Drug Metabolism and Pharmacokinetics

Edited by Mithun Rudrapal

Published in London, United Kingdom

Drug Metabolism and Pharmacokinetics
http://dx.doi.org/10.5772/intechopen.111605
Edited by Mithun Rudrapal

Contributors
Sharad Chand, Manoj S. Dikkatwar, Niharika Pradhan, Urooj Ansari, Gourab Debnath, Vinamra Misra, Ramesh Datta Pant, Priyanka Sharma, Deepali Siwan, Mithun Rudrapal, Dipankar Nath, Dipak Chetia, Yuan Ma, Yihao Zhang, Zefeng Chen, Yuan Tian, Ge Zhang, Tao Zhang, Gaia A. Scalabrino, Neil Frankish, Helen Sheridan, Noor ul Amin Mohsin, Maryam Farrukh, Saba Shahzadi, Muhammad Irfan, Amel Elbasyouni, Dogfounianalo Somda, Stephen Wilson Kpordze, Mercy Jepkorir, Mishell Chantelle Mahora, Jecinta Wanjiru Ndungu, Sally Wambui Kamau, Vera Arthur

First published in London, United Kingdom, 2024 by IntechOpen
IntechOpen is the global imprint of INTECHOPEN LIMITED, registered in England and Wales, registration number: 11086078, 5 Princes Gate Court, London, SW7 2QJ, United Kingdom
Printed in Croatia

British Library Cataloguing-in-Publication Data
A catalogue record for this book is available from the British Library

Additional hard and PDF copies can be obtained from orders@intechopen.com

Drug Metabolism and Pharmacokinetics
Edited by Mithun Rudrapal
p. cm.

This title is part of the Pharmaceutical Science Book Series, Volume 2
Topic: Drug Discovery and Delivery
Series Editor: Rosario Pignatello
Topic Editor: Marilena Vlachou

Print ISBN 978-0-85014-147-4
Online ISBN 978-0-85014-148-1
eBook (PDF) ISBN 978-0-85014-149-8
ISSN 3033-3318

For EU product safety concerns:
IN TECH d.o.o., Prolaz Marije Krucifikse Kozulić 3, 51000 Rijeka, Croatia,
info@intechopen.com or visit our website at intechopen.com.

IntechOpen Book Series
Pharmaceutical Science
Volume 2

Aims and Scope of the Series

Pharmaceutical science focuses on the design, synthesis, formulation, targeting, distribution, safety, and efficacy of active compounds as potential therapeutics. It is a large interdisciplinary discipline that aims to integrate the basic principles of physical and organic chemistry, biochemistry, biology, and engineering to discover, develop, and characterize active compounds and to optimize the formulation and delivery of drugs in the body for offering new and improved safe and efficacious therapies against human diseases. The research areas covered by the pharmaceutical sciences range from medicinal chemistry and pharmaceutical technology to pharmacology and toxicology, which represent the preliminary phases of drug development. Medicinal chemistry involves the design and synthesis of pharmaceuticals as well as the isolation of active agents from natural sources. Computer-aided strategies are increasingly involved in this drug discovery process. Pharmaceutics is a multidisciplinary science that examines the relationships between drug formulation, delivery, distribution, and clinical outcomes. Modern clinical approaches are increasingly relying on controlled release strategies and drug delivery and targeting systems, including nanotechnological platforms (nanomedicine). Pharmacology is the science of drug action in biological systems. Pharmacologists also make drugs as tools to explore aspects of cell and tissue functions. Toxicology is the study of the adverse effects of active agents on living organisms and the ecosystem, including the prevention and amelioration of such adverse effects. This book series includes volumes on Drug Discovery, Delivery, and Pharmacology. Their overall aim is to present the latest research in the whole path of drug discovery and development from different points of view of this multidisciplinary and dynamic field.

Meet the Series Editor

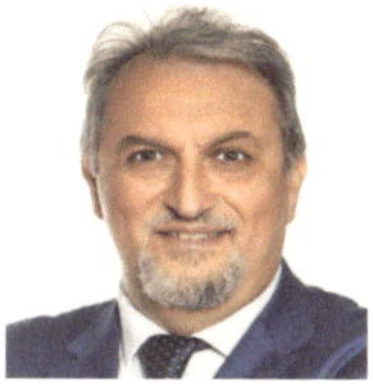

Prof. Rosario Pignatello is a Full Professor of Pharmaceutical Technology and Legislation at the University of Catania, Italy. He is the Director of the Department of Drug and Health Sciences. He has nearly 30 years of experience in the research and development of innovative formulations for the controlled release and targeting of bioactive molecules, through chemical approaches as well as nanotechnological carriers, aimed at treating different disorders. Prof. Pignatello has coauthored about 180 papers and edited a series of textbooks on biomaterials and their application in medicine. The main areas of his research are polymeric and lipid-based micro- and nanoparticles as modified drug delivery systems; vesicular nanocarriers (liposomes, micelles); lipophilic prodrugs and conjugates; synthesis and evaluation of new polymeric biomaterials for drug delivery and tissue regeneration. In particular, Prof. Pignatello works actively in the field of ocular drug delivery, leading the Research Centre for Ocular Nanotechnology, within the NANOMED Centre (Centre for Nanomedicine and Pharmaceutical Nanotechnology) at the University of Catania.

Meet the Volume Editor

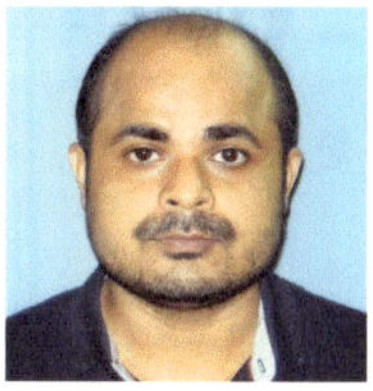

Mithun Rudrapal, Ph.D., FIC, FICS, CChem (India), is an associate professor in the Department of Pharmaceutical Sciences, School of Biotechnology and Pharmaceutical Sciences, Vignan's Foundation for Science, Technology & Research (deemed to be university), Guntur, India. Dr. Rudrapal has been actively engaged in teaching and research in pharmaceutical and allied sciences for more than 14 years. He has more than 1000 publications in peer-reviewed international journals to his credit and has filed several Indian and international patents. In addition, Dr. Rudrapal is the author of a dozen published or forthcoming books. Dr. Rudrapal works in the areas of medicinal chemistry, computer-aided drug design (CADD), drug repurposing, phytochemistry, and dietary polyphenols.

Contents

Preface **XIII**

Section 1
General Aspects **1**

Chapter **3**
Introductory Chapter: Pharmacokinetics and Drug Metabolism with Special Reference to Herbal Formulations
by Priyanka Sharma, Deepali Siwan and Mithun Rudrapal

Chapter 2 **13**
Drug Metabolism: Phase I and Phase II Metabolic Pathways
by Noor ul Amin Mohsin, Maryam Farrukh, Saba Shahzadi and Muhammad Irfan

Chapter 3 **29**
Drug Induced Hematological Disorders: An Undiscussed Stigma
by Sharad Chand, Manoj S. Dikkatwar, Ramesh Datta Pant, Vinamra Misra, Niharika Pradhan, Urooj Ansari and Gourab Debnath

Section 2
Metabolomics and Drug Discovery **45**

Chapter 4 **47**
Metabolomics: Special Emphasis on Basic Drug Discovery and Development
by Dipankar Nath and Dipak Chetia

Chapter 5 **65**
The Role of Bioinformatics in Drug Discovery: A Comprehensive Overview
by Dogfounianalo Somda, Stephen Wilson Kpordze, Mercy Jerpkorir, Mishell Chantelle Mahora, Jecinta Wanjiru Ndungu, Sally Wambui Kamau, Vera Arthur and Amel Elbasyouni

Section 3
Drug Metabolism and Bioanalysis 79

Chapter 6 81
The Modification Strategies for Enhancing the Metabolic Stabilities and Pharmacokinetics of Aptamer Drug Candidates
by Yuan Ma, Yihao Zhang, Zefeng Chen, Yuan Tian and Ge Zhang

Chapter 7 99
Bioactive Indanes: Development and Validation of a Bioanalytical Method of LC-MS/MS for the Determination of PH46A, a New Potential Anti-Inflammatory Agent, in Human Plasma, Urine and Faeces
by Tao Zhang, Gaia A. Scalabrino, Neil Frankish and Helen Sheridan

Preface

Drug metabolism and pharmacokinetics (DMPK) is an important discipline in drug discovery and development programs, which deal with biotransformation and other pharmacokinetic parameters to assess a drug's safety. DMPK basically evaluates a drug's absorption, distribution, metabolism, and excretion (ADME) properties, enabling the discovery and development of a safe and efficacious drug molecule. An understanding of the DMPK process and associated properties is an essential requirement for a candidate drug to become a successful therapeutic agent. Preclinical studies with satisfactory pharmacokinetic, metabolic, and toxicological data reduce failure rates of drug candidates in the clinical phase of drug discovery. Besides adequate potency against the therapeutic target and an acceptable safety profile, a balance of optimized PK properties and minimized drug–drug interactions (DDIs) maximizes the chance of a candidate drug becoming a successful therapeutic agent. In recent times, there has been increased attention on evaluating the pharmacokinetic and safety profile of drug candidates, which includes various pharmacokinetic parameters (aqueous solubility, lipophilicity, cell permeability, bioavailability, protein binding, and metabolism and elimination half-life), DDIs, and toxicokinetics. Various in silico tools and in vitro/in vivo experimental techniques are applied to predict/evaluate such parameters as a rational strategy for the design, optimization, and selection of successful drug candidates. Such studies can help researchers and drug developers predict potential risks of failure early in drug development, as well as provide pre-clinical evidence to conduct clinical trials.

Mithun Rudrapal
Department of Pharmaceutical Sciences,
School of Biotechnology and Pharmaceutical Sciences,
Vignan's Foundation for Science, Technology and Research (Deemed to be University),
Guntur, India

Section 1

General Aspects

Chapter

Introductory Chapter: Pharmacokinetics and Drug Metabolism with Special Reference to Herbal Formulations

Priyanka Sharma, Deepali Siwan and Mithun Rudrapal

1. Introduction to herbal formulations

Plant-based treatments are crucial in achieving Sustainable Development Goal 3 (SDG 3) to ensure healthy lives and promote well-being. Integrating effective and safe herbal medical systems with traditional pharmaceutical systems can significantly enhance essential healthcare services. A survey conducted in Germany revealed that various age groups opt for herbal remedies due to dissatisfaction with allopathic treatments, the synergistic effects of medicinal plants, historical usage, and unique knowledge [1]. In the face of emerging diseases like SARS-COV-2 and mycosis, interest in phytotherapy has been rekindled to strengthen the healthcare system and combat the ongoing epidemic. Immunity-boosting plants, herbal remedies, and AYUSH compositions are being considered as preventive measures. Specific botanical formulations include the aqueous solution of Guduchi and pippali, AYUSH 64, and Guduchi aq. extracts have shown promise for mild to moderate and asymptomatic COVID-19 patients [2]. Ashwagandha and Guduchi extracts are also recommended for preventive use against COVID-19, with Withaferin A potentially acting as a therapeutic agent to inhibit viral spread. However, further research is needed to determine the long-term safety and optimal dosage [3]. Currently, herbal medicines straddle the line between conventional drugs and food. This chapter elucidates their historical significance, integration into modern healthcare, and metabolic and pharmacokinetic profiles within the human body.

1.1 Importance of understanding herbal formulations' metabolism and pharmacokinetics

Researchers are increasingly curious about the impact of herbal formulations on metabolism and pharmacokinetics. Pharmacokinetics (PK), a newly developed approach, is instrumental in studying drug absorption, distribution, metabolism, and excretion in vivo. When combined with other techniques, PK helps determine the active components of medicinal plants [4–6]. Pharmacokinetic measures like biological half-life, clearance, and AUC reveal dynamic processes of these components in vivo. Contrasting pharmacokinetic parameters aids in understanding their characteristics [7, 8]. This has three benefits: precise explanation of herbal formulation effects

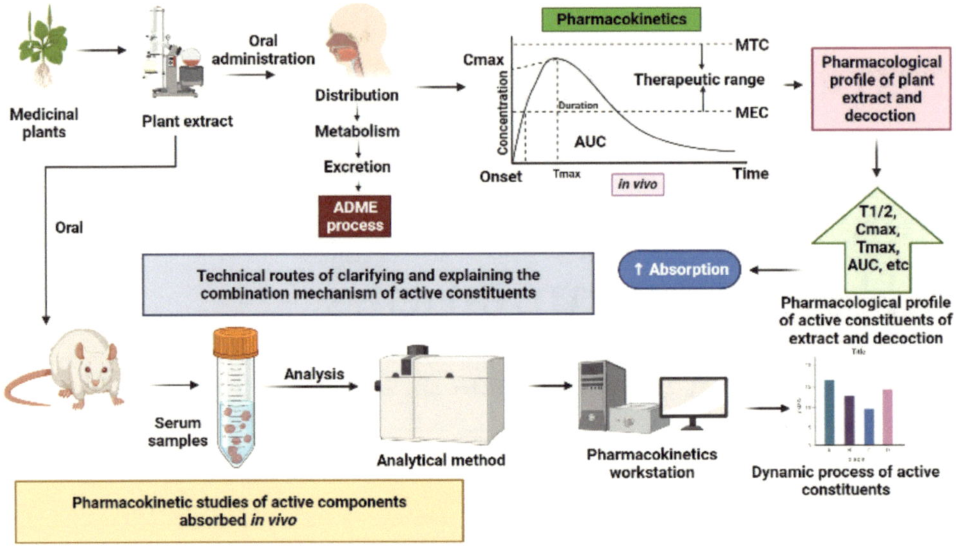

Figure 1.
Representation of pharmacokinetics studies of active constituents via in vivo. Cmax, maximum plasma concentration; MTC, minimum toxic concentration; Tmax, time to Cmax; AUC, area under curve; MEC, minimum effective concentration.

by identifying components, clarifying interactions of active substances (**Figure 1**), and demonstrating dynamic actions of active ingredients in vivo (**Figure 1**). These discoveries support the clinical use and understanding of medicinal plants.

Researchers discovered how the active components in medicinal plants produce their therapeutic benefits by thoroughly examining them. For instance, artemisinin was employed as a malaria preventative. Rhein, geniposide, and 6,7-dimethylesculetin were successful treatments for hepatic damage syndrome. Nonbacterial prostatitis was treated with berberine. Additionally, research employing PK has helped us to better understand the dynamic mechanisms of the active components of medicinal plants in vivo [2, 3], shown in **Figure 1**.

2. Absorption, distribution, metabolism, and excretion (ADME) of herbal compounds

2.1 Absorption of herbal compounds in the gastrointestinal tract

The impact of oral herbal therapies on individuals and their influencing factors remains understudied. Oral absorption is critical for defining bioavailability of medicinal ingredients from plants. Research on oral absorption is primarily based on animal and cell studies (e.g., Caco-2 cells). Some herbal substances have been assessed for oral bioavailability values, influenced by factors such as gastric fluid solubility, membrane permeability, gastrointestinal tract deprivation, and transporters like P-glycoprotein (P-gp/MDR1/ABCB1). Low or weak intestinal absorption may lead to inadequate oral bioavailability of herbal ingredients, as seen with curcumin. To enhance bioavailability, various formulations like liposomes and nanotechnology-based approaches have been developed [9]. Further research is needed to optimize oral herbal therapies and maximize their therapeutic potential.

2.2 Distribution of herbal compounds in the body

The albumin from human serum (HSA), 1-acid glycoprotein (AGP), lipoprotein, or and globulin are examples of plasma proteins connected to the ADME and pharmacodynamics properties of drugs in the body through bidirectional interactions.

The hydrophobic cavity in HSA is crucial in explaining how it affects the distribution and efficacy of medications. The hydrophobic cavity in HSA can alter the distribution of cells in vivo and in vitro and increase the apparent dissolution of hydrophobic drugs in plasma.

Human serum albumin and berberine, a conventional herbal remedy used to treat gastrointestinal diseases, were examined by Hu et al. The findings showed that the hydrophobic pocket of subdomain IIA was where berberine bound most frequently and that electrostatic forces played a significant role in the interaction of berberine and HSA.

The blood–brain barrier (BBB), which blocks substances from circulating blood from entering the brain through paracellular and transcellular routes, comprises humans' tightly connected brain endothelial cells. These multidrug transporters can prevent harmful circulatory chemicals, including herbal medicines, from making it to the brain. However, these transporters will impede and lessen the efficiency of herbal drugs that impact the central nervous system [10].

2.3 Metabolism of herbal compounds in the liver

The human gut is where herbal substances are subjected to CYP- and UGT-mediated metabolism, which may be a critical factor in influencing intake and bioavailability. Following oral ingestion, herbal essences are vulnerable to presystemic oxidative and/or coupling metabolism, and the presence of several CYPs (in particular CYP3A4), and UGTs is significant in the gut. When absorbing diverse herbal compounds from the core, intestinal CYP3A4 can act as a very effective metabolic barrier without the help of the liver.

Numerous herbal substances often undergo intestinal hydrolysis, yielding pharmacologically active or degraded metabolites. Many herbal treatments' glycosides typically undergo intestinal deglycosylation before being absorbed, and phenolic compounds' aglycones are then sulfated or glucuronidated in the gut and liver. Emodin and sennidin are broken down in the colon to create their pharmacologically effective aglycones [11].

2.4 Excretion of herbal compounds from the body

Herbal medicines taken orally undergo absorption, metabolism, and subsequent elimination through feces and/or kidneys. Most plant natural products have a short elimination half-life, and their parent chemicals or metabolites can be detected in urine and feces. Urinary excretion is the primary route for eliminating herbal medicine metabolites or parent chemicals, followed by biliary excretion, involving specific drug transporters. For instance, after intravenous administration of 100 mg quercetin, 7.4% was excreted in the urine as a conjugation metabolite, and 0.65% remained unchanged. Quercetin and kaempferol showed recovery rates of 99.7% and 97.4%, respectively. Many herbal medicines are also eliminated through biliary excretion, with fecal recovery rates varying depending on the compound administered [12–16]. The exact role of hepatic transporters in biliary elimination of herbal treatments remains uncertain.

3. Enzymes involved in the metabolism of herbal compounds

Enzymes play a crucial role in the metabolism of herbal compounds, impacting their absorption, distribution, and elimination within the body. Phase I enzymes, such as Cytochrome P450 (CYP) and Flavin-Containing Monooxygenases (FMO), initiate biotransformation reactions like oxidation, reduction, and hydrolysis. These reactions can either enhance or reduce the biological activity of herbal compounds. Phase II enzymes, like Glucuronosyltransferases, Sulfotransferases, and Glutathione S-Transferases, facilitate conjugation reactions, making herbal compounds more water-soluble for easier excretion [17]. The interplay between Phase I and Phase II enzymes influences the fate of herbal compounds, affecting their pharmacokinetics, efficacy, and potential interactions with other drugs. Understanding these enzyme-mediated processes is crucial for optimizing the therapeutic use of herbal formulations and ensuring patient safety.

3.1 Cytochrome P450 enzymes and herbal drug metabolism

Cytochrome P450 (CYP) enzymes are a group of heme-containing proteins primarily found in the liver and other tissues. They play a crucial role in metabolizing a diverse range of drugs, including herbal compounds. In the metabolism of herbal drugs, CYP enzymes are responsible for transforming the active constituents present in herbal formulations. This biotransformation involves various chemical reactions such as oxidation, hydroxylation, and dealkylation, leading to the formation of metabolites with different pharmacological properties than the original compounds [18]. Consequently, the activity of CYP enzymes can significantly impact the efficacy, safety, and potential interactions of herbal drugs with other medications. It is crucial for healthcare professionals and researchers to understand the role of CYP enzymes in herbal drug metabolism to optimize therapies and ensure patient safety when using herbal formulations in combination with conventional medicines.

3.2 Glucuronidation and other phase II enzymes

Glucuronidation is a significant Phase II biotransformation reaction responsible for metabolizing herbal compounds and other xenobiotics. UDP-glucuronosyltransferases (UGTs) are the enzymes involved in this process, transferring glucuronic acid from UDP-glucuronic acid to the functional groups of herbal compounds, increasing their hydrophilicity and facilitating their excretion from the body. Other important Phase II enzymes in herbal drug metabolism include sulfotransferases, methyltransferases, and glutathione S-transferases (GSTs). Sulfotransferases add sulfate groups, methyltransferases add methyl groups, and GSTs conjugate herbal compounds with glutathione, promoting detoxification and enhanced excretion. The interplay of Phase II enzymes complements Phase I reactions, ensuring efficient and safe herbal compound metabolism [19]. Understanding these enzymatic processes is crucial for optimizing herbal formulations' use and promoting their safe integration into healthcare practices.

3.3 Transporters and their role in herbal drug interactions

Transporters are membrane proteins that play a crucial role in the absorption, distribution, and elimination of herbal compounds and other drugs in the body.

Table 1 provides examples of herbal compounds and their interactions with transporters, illustrating the impact on the pharmacokinetics of co-administered drugs. The table likely includes information about specific herbal blends, their respective transporters, and their effects on the absorption, distribution, and elimination of other drugs. These examples showcase how herbal formulations can influence the activity of transporters, leading to altered drug bioavailability and potential herb-drug interactions [20]. Understanding such interactions is crucial for healthcare professionals to ensure the safe and effective use of herbal and conventional drugs.

Enzymes	Examples	Function
Phase I enzymes	Cytochrome P450 (CYP) enzymes	Oxidation, Reduction, and Hydrolysis of herbal compounds into more water-soluble metabolites.
	Flavin-containing monooxygenases (FMOs)	Involved in the oxidation of nitrogen, sulfur, and phosphorous-containing compounds.
Phase II enzymes	UDP-glucuronosyltransferases (UGTs)	Conjugation of herbal compounds with glucuronic acid, increasing water solubility for excretion.
	Sulfotransferases (SULTs)	Conjugation of herbal compounds with sulfate, enhances their excretion.
	Glutathione S-transferases (GSTs)	Conjugation of herbal compounds with glutathione facilitates their elimination.
	N-Acetyltransferases (NATs)	Conjugation of herbal compounds with acetyl groups, promoting excretion.
Cytochrome P450 (CYP) enzymes	CYP3A4	Metabolizes a wide range of herbal compounds and drugs commonly involved in interactions.
	CYP2D6	Metabolizes several herbal compounds and drugs, and genetic polymorphisms may affect metabolism.
	CYP2C9	Metabolizes various herbal compounds and drugs, which is important in drug interactions.
Transporters	P-glycoprotein (P-gp)	Efflux transporter pumps herbal compounds out of cells, affecting absorption and distribution.
	Multidrug Resistance-Associated Proteins (MRPs)	Efflux transporters are involved in herbal compounds and drug elimination.
	Breast Cancer Resistance Protein (BCRP)	Efflux transporter limiting absorption and distribution of herbal compounds and drugs.
	Organic Anion Transporting Polypeptides (OATPs)	Uptake transporters facilitate herbal compound absorption into cells.
	Organic Cation Transporters (OCTs)	Uptake transporters involved in the cellular uptake of herbal compounds

Table 1.
The examples of enzymes, cytochrome P450 enzymes, and transporters involved in the metabolism and interactions of herbal compounds.

Integrating this knowledge into clinical practice can enhance patient outcomes and minimize the risk of adverse effect.

4. Factors affecting pharmacokinetics of herbal formulations

The Pharmacokinetics of herbal formulations is affected by chemical composition, the bioavailability of active compounds, formulation methods, and individual variability in metabolism, genetics, age, and health status. Drug interactions and co-administration with other substances also influence the pharmacokinetic profile, necessitating safe and effective clinical use consideration.

4.1 Herb-drug interactions and their impact on pharmacokinetics

Herb-drug interactions occur when herbal compounds interact with conventional medications, affecting their pharmacokinetics. These interactions can lead to altered drug absorption, distribution, metabolism, or excretion, potentially impacting therapeutic outcomes or causing adverse effects. Understanding and monitoring such interactions are crucial in clinical settings to ensure the safe and effective use of both herbal remedies and pharmaceutical drugs. Healthcare professionals must be vigilant in assessing and managing herb-drug interactions to optimize patient outcomes and safety [21].

4.2 Influence of genetics and individual variation on herbal drug metabolism

Genetics and individual variation play a crucial role in herbal drug metabolism. Genetic polymorphisms in drug-metabolizing enzymes and drug transporters can lead to significant inter-individual differences in how herbal compounds are processed and eliminated from the body. Variations in these genes can affect the efficacy and safety of

Dietary component	Effect on herbal drug absorption
High-fat foods	May increase the absorption of lipophilic herbal compounds.
High-fiber foods	Can delay the absorption of herbal drugs and reduce their bioavailability.
Grapefruit juice	Can inhibit the activity of certain drug-metabolizing enzymes, affecting drug absorption.
Alcohol	May enhance the absorption of some herbal compounds and alter drug metabolism.
Calcium-rich foods	Can interfere with the absorption of certain herbal drugs.
Caffeine	May enhance the absorption of certain herbal compounds.
Spices and Piperine	Piperine present in black pepper can increase the bioavailability of herbal drugs.
Probiotics	Can influence the gut microbiota and affect the metabolism of herbal compounds.
Iron-rich foods	May reduce the absorption of certain herbal drugs.

Table 2.
Effect of food and dietary components on herbal drug absorption [22, 23].

herbal formulations and contribute to herb-drug interactions. Pharmacogenomic studies help identify genetic factors influencing herbal drug metabolism, enabling personalized treatment approaches. Considering individual genetic variations is essential to optimize herbal therapy, minimize adverse reactions, and achieve desired therapeutic outcomes for each patient. Moreover, the Effect of Food and Dietary Components on Herbal Drug Absorption is preciously discussed in **Table 2**.

5. Conclusion

The chapter emphasizes the importance of understanding the dynamic processes by which herbal compounds are absorbed, distributed, metabolized, and excreted in the body. Researchers are increasingly exploring the impact of herbal formulations on metabolism and pharmacokinetics using pharmacokinetic (PK) studies. PK helps identify active components, elucidate the effects of herbal formulations, and understand their dynamic actions in vivo. Chemical composition, bioavailability, formulation methods, and individual variability in metabolism and genetics influence herbal drug metabolism. The chapter also discusses herb-drug interactions, the role of enzymes and transporters, and the effect of food and dietary components on herbal drug absorption. Understanding these processes is crucial for optimizing herbal therapies and ensuring safe and effective integration into healthcare practices.

Conflict of interest

The authors declare no conflict of interest.

Author details

Priyanka Sharma[1], Deepali Siwan[1] and Mithun Rudrapal[2]*

1 Department of Pharmacology, Delhi Pharmaceutical Sciences and Research University, Delhi, India

2 Department of Pharmaceutical Sciences, School of Biotechnology and Pharmaceutical Sciences, Vignan's Foundation for Science, Technology and Research (Deemed to be University), Guntur, India

*Address all correspondence to: rsmrpal@gmail.com

References

[1] Welz AN, Emberger-Klein A, Menrad K. Why people use herbal medicine: Insights from a focus-group study in Germany. BMC Complementary and Alternative Medicine. 2018;**18**:1-9

[2] Chaturvedi S, Kumar N, Tillu G, Deshpande S, Patwardhan B. AYUSH, modern medicine and the Covid-19 pandemic. Indian Journal of Medical Ethics. 2020;**5**(03):191-195

[3] Straughn AR, Kakar SS. Withaferin a: A potential therapeutic agent against COVID-19 infection. Journal of Ovarian Research. 2020;**13**(1):79

[4] Sun H, Wu F, Zhang A, Wei W, Han Y, Wang X. Pharmacokinetic study of schisandrin, schisandrol B, schisantherin a, deoxyschisandrin, and schisandrin B in rat plasma after oral administration of S hengmaisan formula by UPLC-MS. Journal of Separation Science. 2013;**36**(3):485-491

[5] Sun H, Dong T, Zhang A, Yang J, Yan G, Sakurai T, et al. Pharmacokinetics of hesperetin and naringenin in the Zhi Zhu wan, a traditional Chinese medicinal formulae, and its pharmacodynamics study. Phytotherapy Research. 2013;**27**(9):1345-1351

[6] Zhang AH, Sun H, Han Y, Yan GL, Yuan Y, Song GC, et al. Ultraperformance liquid chromatography–mass spectrometry based comprehensive metabolomics combined with pattern recognition and network analysis methods for characterization of metabolites and metabolic pathways from biological data sets. Analytical Chemistry. 2013;**85**(15):7606-7612

[7] Li QJ, Zhang AH, Sun H, Wang XJ. Pharmacokinetics applications of traditional Chinese medicines. World Journal of Traditional Chinese Medicine. 2016;**2**(1):42-47

[8] Sharma RA, McLelland HR, Hill KA, Ireson CR, Euden SA, Manson MM, et al. Pharmacodynamic and pharmacokinetic study of oral curcuma extract in patients with colorectal cancer. Clinical Cancer Research. 2001;**7**(7):1894-1900

[9] Zhang W, Yang S, He H, Liu C, Chen W, Tang X. Technology for improving the bioavailability of small molecules extracted from traditional Chinese medicines. Expert Opinion on Drug Delivery. 2009;**6**(11):1247-1259

[10] Banker MJ, Clark TH. Plasma/ serum protein binding determinations. Current Drug Metabolism. 2008;**9**(9):854-859

[11] Alrefai WA, Gill RK. Bile acid transporters: Structure, function, regulation and pathophysiological implications. Pharmaceutical Research. 2007;**24**:1803-1823

[12] Gugler R, Leschik M, Dengler HJ. Disposition of quercetin in man after single oral and intravenous doses. European Journal of Clinical Pharmacology. 1975;**9**(2-3):229-234

[13] Löscher W, Potschka H. Blood-brain barrier active efflux transporters: ATP-binding cassette gene family. NeuroRx. 2005;**2**(1):86-98

[14] Hawkins BT, Davis TP. The blood-brain barrier/neurovascular unit in health and disease. Pharmacological Reviews. 2005;**57**(2):173-85.76

[15] Borst P, Elferink RO. Mammalian ABC transporters in health and disease.

Annual Review of Biochemistry. 2002;**71**:537-592

[16] Zhou SF, Wang LL, Di YM, Xue CC, Duan W, Li CG, et al. Substrates and inhibitors of human multidrug resistance associated proteins and the implications in drug development. Current Mmedicinal Chemistry. 2008;**15**(20):1981-2039

[17] Pang X, Tang C, Guo R, Therapeutics XCP. Non-cytochrome P450 enzymes involved in the oxidative metabolism of xenobiotics: Focus on the regulation of gene expression and enzyme activity. Pharmacology and Therapeutics. 2022;**233**:108020

[18] Schneider E, Bioelectronics DC-B. Cytochrome P450 (CYP) enzymes and the development of CYP biosensors. Biosensors and Bioelectronics. 2013;**39**(1):1-13

[19] Mazerska Z, Mróz A, MP-P. The role of glucuronidation in drug resistance. Pharmacology and Therapeutics. 2016;**159**:35-55

[20] Wu X, Ma J, Ye Y, BL-J of C. Transporter modulation by Chinese herbal medicines and its mediated pharmacokinetic herb-drug interactions. Journal Chromatography B Analytical Technologies in the Biomedical Life Sciences. 2016;**1026**:236-253

[21] Mukherjee P, RH--based validation of herbal. Bioavailability of herbal products: Approach toward improved pharmacokinetics. Elsevier. 2015

[22] Cheng W, Xia K, Wu S, Li Y. Herb-drug interactions and their impact on pharmacokinetics: An update. Current Drug Metabolism. 2023;**24**(1):28-69

[23] Anderson KE. Effects of specific foods and dietary components on drug metabolism. In: Boullata JI, Armenti VT, editors. Handbook of DrugNutrient Interactions. New York: Humana Press; 2009. pp. 243-265

Chapter 2

Drug Metabolism: Phase I and Phase II Metabolic Pathways

Noor ul Amin Mohsin, Maryam Farrukh, Saba Shahzadi and Muhammad Irfan

Abstract

Drug metabolism comprises the metabolism of endogenous and exogenous substances. During metabolism most drugs lose the pharmacological activity and are excreted from the body. Drug metabolic reactions are divided into two classes i.e. phase I and phase II metabolic reactions. The characterisation of drug metabolising enzyme is necessary in order to determine the toxic metabolites of drugs. The understanding of drug metabolism is essential for new drug design and development. The evaluation of pharmacokinetic properties is necessary to see whether they can be useful drug candidates. In this chapter we have discussed drug metabolic reaction and drug metabolising enzymes with the help of examples of drug molecules.

Keywords: cytochrome p450, glucuronic acid, glutathione, prodrug, toxic metabolites, drug design

1. Introduction

The human body is exposed to various foreign particles that are dust particles, food, toxins, and air pollutants. These foreign particles are collectively called xenobiotics. The term xeno means foreign, which is not a part of our body normally. When these foreign particles enter the body, the body has a mechanism to modify these particles so that they are excreted from the body. This process is called metabolism. Drugs are also regarded as xenobiotics as drugs are foreign particles. The process of drug metabolism is also called biotransformation. Normally, the metabolism decreases pharmacological effect but sometimes metabolism produces toxic metabolites or active metabolites. Drugs which undergo metabolism to produce a pharmacological effect are called prodrugs. Some drugs undergo metabolism to produce toxic metabolites that are carcinogenic or mutagenic. The liver is the main site of metabolism in the body. Some drugs are metabolised before reaching the systemic circulation, this is called the first-pass effect. Drug metabolism also occurs in the kidney, skin and gastrointestinal tract (GIT) etc. There are two phases of drug metabolism i.e. phase I metabolic reactions and phase II metabolic reactions.

2. Phase I reaction

These are non-synthetic reactions that introduce a hydrophilic group or unmask the already present hydrophilic group in these drugs. Phase I reactions include oxidation, reduction and hydrolysis.

2.1 Oxidation

The process of oxidation is catalysed by a class of enzymes that are collectively called cytochrome P450 (Cyp-450). They are present in the smooth endoplasmic reticulum (SER) of the liver. These are also known as microsomal enzymes because they are present in the microsome of SER [1]. The Cyp-450 consists of a protoporphyrin ring (**Figure 1**) having four (4) pyrrole rings. Pyrrole is a five-membered heterocyclic ring which contains one nitrogen atom. In Cyp450, four pyrrole rings are linked by a methylene bridge and the nitrogen of each pyrrole ring are combined with iron. The iron is present in ferric form (Fe^{+3}) and is also associated with the sulphur of cysteine which is the peptide part. It can form a complex with carbon monoxide (CO). The complex of ferric (Fe^{+3}) with CO gives an absorption bond at 450 nm wavelength hence these enzymes are called CYP-450 [2].

Various drugs undergo the process of oxidation. In oxidation, first of all, the drug is attached to CYP-450 to form a complex. The iron in CYP-450 is converted into a ferrous form. It gains an electron and this reaction is catalysed by CYP-450 reductase and functions with a co-enzyme that is nicotinamide adenine dinucleotide phosphate hydrogenase (NADPH) shifts an electron from co-enzyme to iron (CYP-P450). In the next step, molecular oxygen gets attached to the complex of the drug and CYP450. The oxygen attached to the complex is converted into activated oxygen by a series of steps. The iron loses an electron and is converted into a ferric form by CYP-450

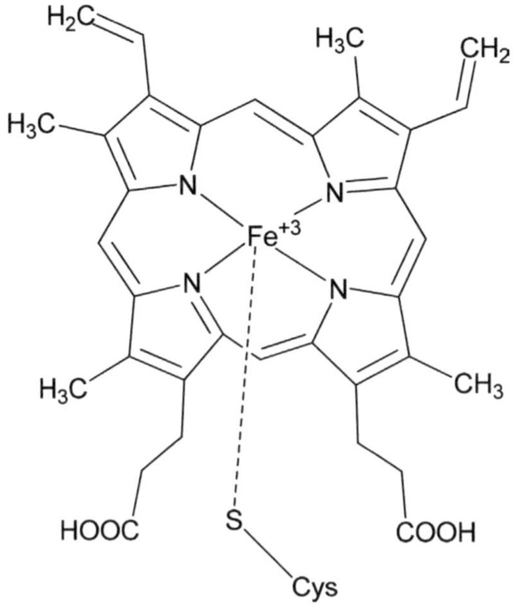

Figure 1.
Porphyrin ring of cytochrome P450.

reductase and NADPH. The molecular oxygen is converted into atomic oxygen in the process of oxidation. One atom of oxygen is converted into the water molecule and another atom of oxygen is incorporated into the xenobiotic. CYP-450 again comes in its original form and the drug molecule is oxidised. There are many types and sub-types of CYP450 but the most important are CYP1A2, CYP2C9, CYP2D6, CYP2A6, CYP2E1, and CYP3A4. This system is non-specific and catalyses the oxidation of a large number of drugs. Lipid soluble substances are excellent substrates of this system because these enzymes are located mainly in lipid tissues. The process of oxidation takes place at different functional groups and hetero atoms. For example, aromatic rings, the alkyl group and the amino group [3]. This process takes place in drugs which contain aromatic rings in their structures. The hydrophilic group is introduced in the aromatic ring. This mostly occurs at the para position via the formation of an epoxide intermediate. For example, the conversion of acetanilide into acetaminophen (**Figure 2**) is an example of aromatic hydroxylation.

Some drug molecules contain heteroatom in their structure and the process of oxidation takes place at the heteroatom. Sulphur heteroatoms are oxidised to sulf-oxides (**Figure 3**) and sulfones. Secondary amines are converted into lactam. Flavin monooxygenase (FMO) catalyses oxidation in drugs that contain hetero atoms in their structure. In this case, first of all, activation of molecular oxygen takes place before the attachment of xenobiotics but in the CYP-450 enzyme, the first step involves the attachment of the drug and then activation of molecular oxygen. For example, the anticancer agent tamoxifen is converted into tamoxifen N-oxide by FMO [4].

The alkyl groups are removed from the amino group by the process of oxidation. Tertiary amines are converted to secondary amines and secondary amines are converted to primary amines. The rate of N-dealkylation depends upon the chain length of the alkyl group [5]. Mephorbarbital has a tertiary amine and it is converted

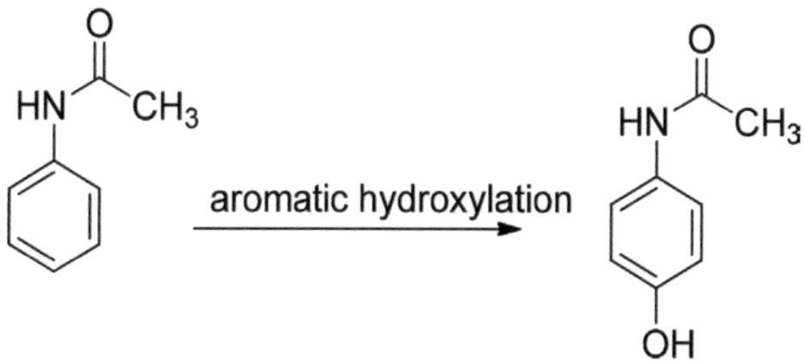

Figure 2.
Conversion of acetanilide into acetaminophen.

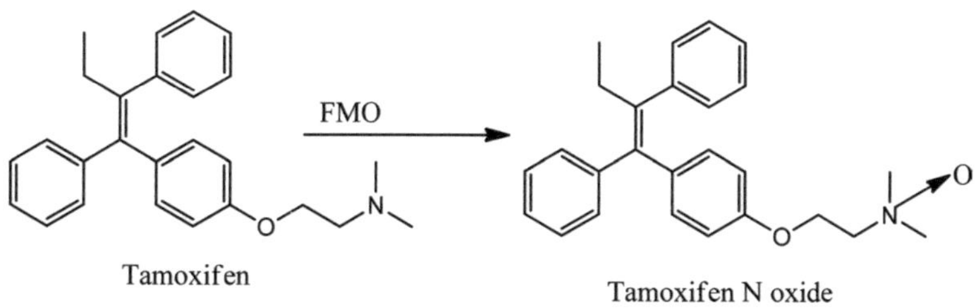

Figure 3.
Oxidation of tamoxifen into tamoxifen N-oxide.

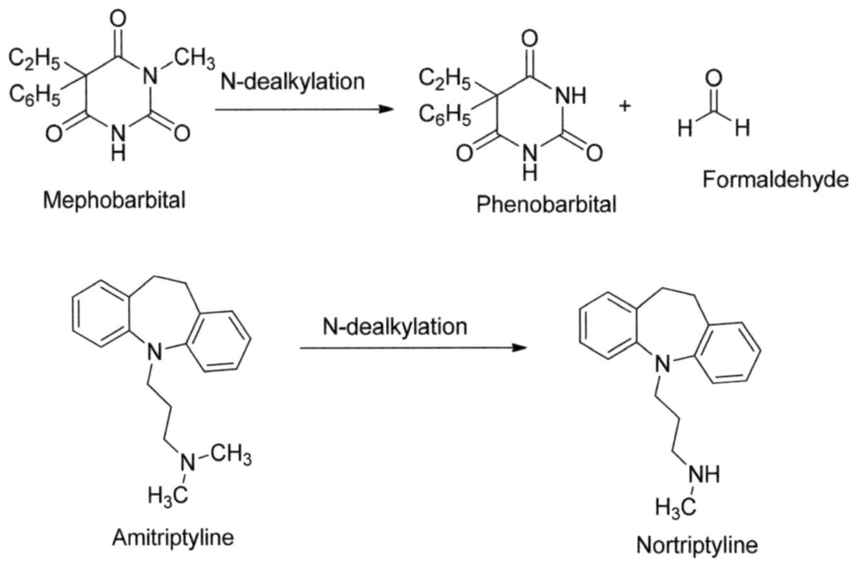

Figure 4.
Examples of n-dealkylation.

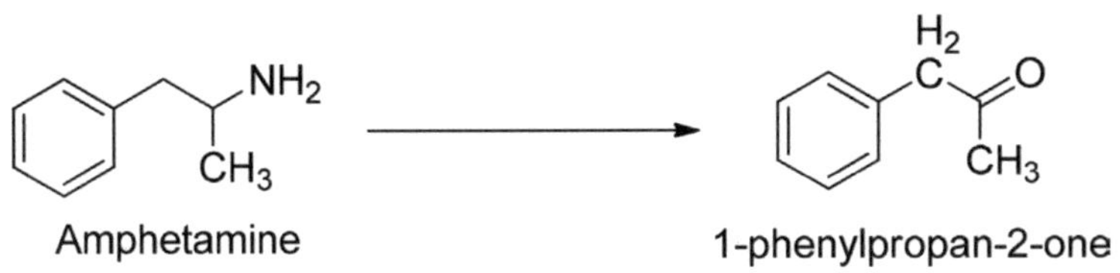

Figure 5.
Deamination of amphetamine into phenylpropanone.

into phenobarbital which has a secondary amine (**Figure 4**). The methyl group is converted into formaldehyde. Primary amines are more water solubility than secondary and tertiary amines. Usually, drugs lose pharmacological activity after oxidation but phenobarbital retains its activity after oxidation. The n-dealkylation produces a pharmacologically active compound. The conversion of amitriptyline into nortriptyline is also an example of n-dealkylation.

Drugs molecules that contain a primary amino (NH_2) group undergo oxidative deamination (**Figure 5**) in which the amino group is directly removed and oxygen is incorporated in drug molecules. Ammonia (NH_3) is converted into uric acid that is excreted from the body via urine.

Drug molecules having ether linkage in their structure undergo the process of oxidative dealkylation. An alkyl group is removed from oxygen in compounds that undergo oxidation dealkylation. For example, the conversion of phenacetin into acetaminophen (**Figure 6**).

The hydrophilic group (-OH) has been unmasked in acetaminophen at this site. Phenacetin has also analgesic and antipyretic activity but due to hepatotoxicity toxicity, it was withdrawn from the market. But it was proved that phenacetin is converted into acetaminophen in the body by oxidative dealkylation which is a safer drug than phenacetin.

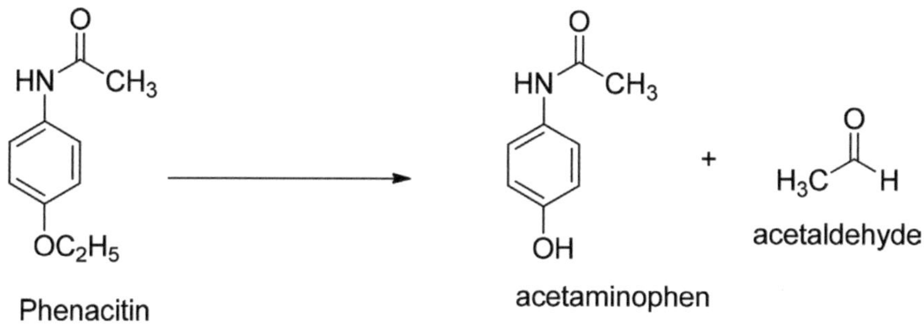

Figure 6.
Oxidative dealkylation of phenacitin into acetaminophen.

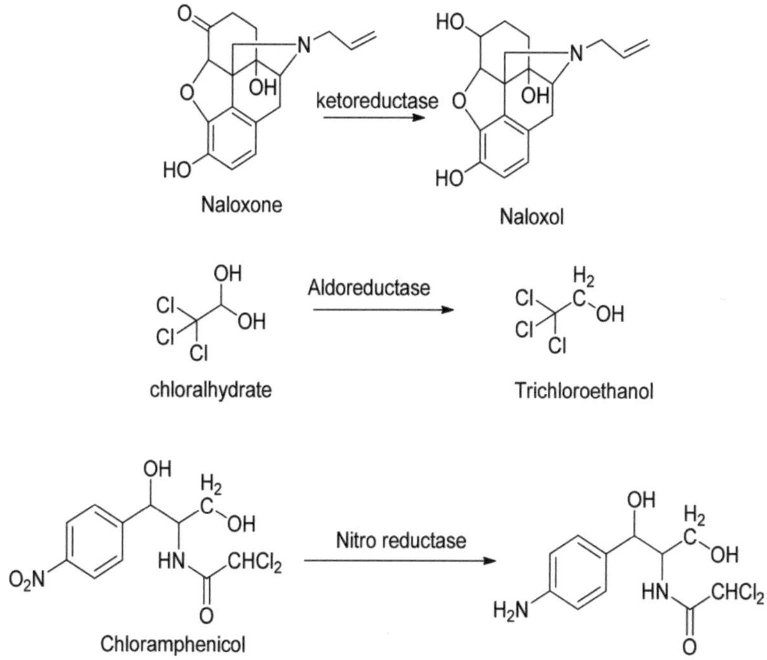

Figure 7.
Nitro and aldo reduction of chloramphenicol and chloral hydrate.

2.2 Reduction

Drug molecules which contain reducible groups like nitro, azo, alkene, aldehydes, and ketones easily undergo the process of reduction. The process of reduction is catalysed by specific enzymes which catalyse the reduction for specific classes. The nitro reductase is required for the reduction of the nitro group. The azo reductase is required for the reduction of the azo group. Aldo-keto reductases are required for the reduction of aldehydes and ketones. Opiate antagonist naloxone is reduced in liver to naloxol. Chloral hydrate undergoes the process of reduction and is converted into trichloroethanol (**Figure 7**). These enzymes are mainly located in the liver but small quantities are present in lungs and kidney. The enzymes which carry out the process of reduction also require a co-enzyme NADPH (nicotinamide adenine dinucleotide

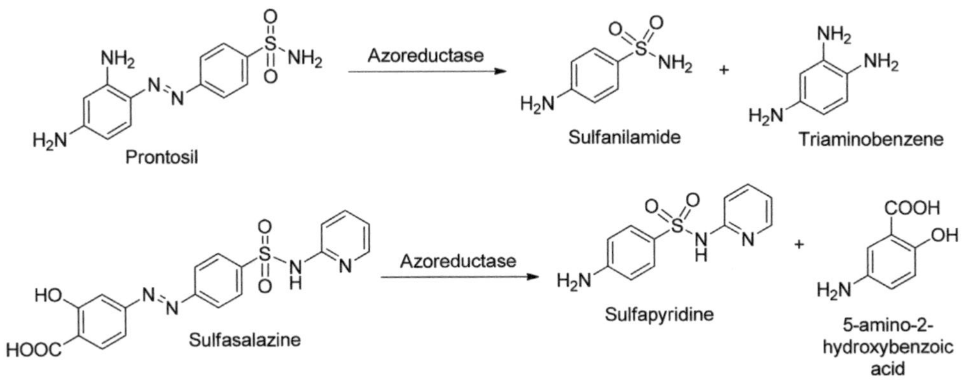

Figure 8.
Azo reduction of prontosil and sulfasalazine.

phosphate hydrogenase) [6]. The reduction introduces a hydrophilic group in the drug molecule or unmasks the already present hydrophilic group. The metabolism of chloramphenicol is an example of nitro reduction. It is an antibiotic and a protein synthesis inhibitor. It contains the nitro (-NO_2) group, reduction takes place in this group and it is converted into the amino (-NH_2) group and the remaining structure is the same.

Certain drugs contain azo group in their structures, for example, prontosil. The azo group is reduced and converted into two fragments sulfanilamide and triaminobenzene (**Figure 8**). Sulfanilamide is a prototype sulphonamide used as an antibacterial agent. Azo reductases are present in the liver. Sulfasalazine is a sulfonamide derivative used in ulcerative colitis. It is a prodrug and carries azo linkage that reduces in the intestine to form sulfapyridine and p-amino salicylic acid. Sulfpyridine has antibacterial activity. This process of reduction is catalysed by bacteria present in the intestines (normal intestinal flora) which produce the enzyme [7].

2.3 Hydrolysis

The process of hydrolysis takes place in drug molecules which contain ester or amide linkage in their structure. Drug molecules like acetylcholine, suxamethonium, acetylsalicylic acid and procaine carry ester linkage in their scaffolds (**Figure 9**).

Aspirin is an acid but also contains an ester group in its structure. The ester group is hydrolysed. Esterases and pseudocholinesterase are enzymes which catalyse the process of hydrolysis of the drugs-containing ester groups. Esterases are specific in its action but pseudocholinesterase is not specific in their action. Pseudocholinesterases have broad specificity and can catalyse various groups. The hydrolysis of amides is catalysed by amidases, and peptidases. Procaine is a local anaesthetic and also contains an ester linkage. When the ester group is hydrolysed, acid and alcohol are formed. Diethylamino ethanol and p-aminobenzoic acid are products of the hydrolysis of procaine. The hydroxyl group is highly hydrophilic so the drug undergoes the process of phase II metabolism readily. The hydrolysis of drugs containing the amide group is very slow while the hydrolysis of the ester group is faster [8]. Chloramphenicol has a bitter taste so combined with palmitic acid to produce chloramphenicol palmitate (**Figure 10**). This prodrug is in ester form and then after absorption in the systemic circulation, this ester form of chloramphenicol undergoes hydrolysis and releases an active drug that is chloramphenicol.

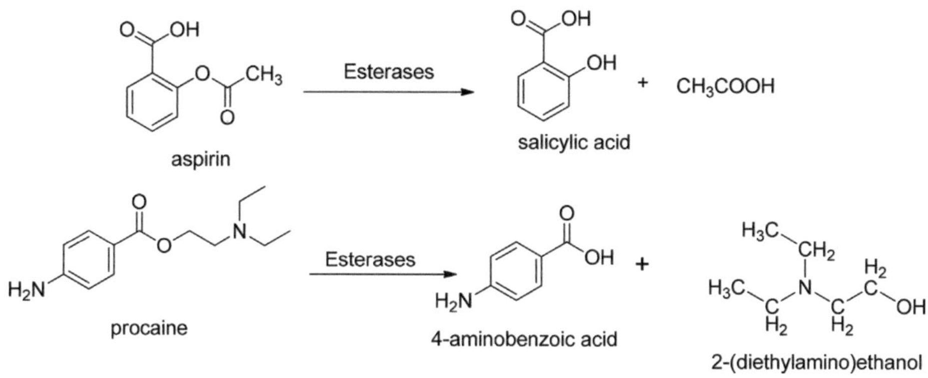

Figure 9.
Ester hydrolysis of aspirin and procaine.

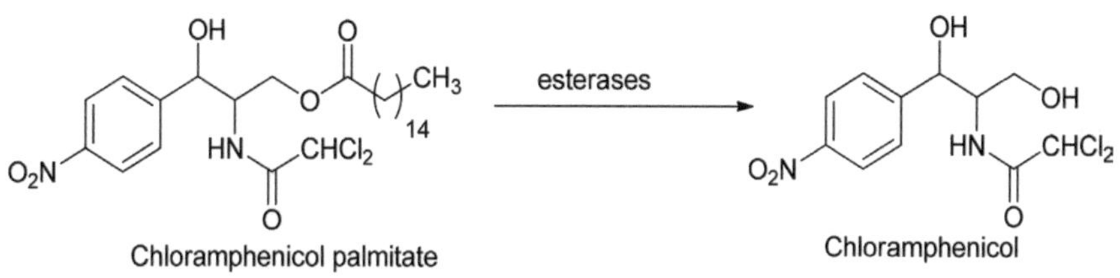

Figure 10.
Ester hydrolysis of chloramphenicol palmitate.

Therefore, esters are presented as prodrug form and amides can be presented as a slow-release drug.

3. Phase II metabolism

Phase II metabolic reactions represents the most important metabolic reaction and are called synthetic reactions. In phase II metabolic reactions, an endogenous molecule is attached to a drug molecule. Endogenous molecules are hydrophilic and increase the hydrophilicity of the drug. Phase II metabolic reactions decrease the affinity of the drug with the receptor and they are excreted from the body. The phase II reactions are collectively called conjugation reactions. Glucuronic acid conjugation, sulfate conjugation, amino acid conjugation, glutathione conjugation, acetylation, methylation are different types of phase II metabolic reactions. Phase II metabolic reactions are not substrate-specific. At one functional group, more than one conjugating enzymes can act. For example, the hydroxyl group can undergo glucuronic acid conjugation, sulfate conjugation and acetylation reactions. The amino group can be metabolised by glucuronic acid conjugation and acetylation.

3.1 Glucuronic acid conjugation

Glucuronic acid is an oxidation product of glucose and is a hydrophilic molecule. In this reaction, the molecule of glucuronic acid becomes attached to the drug molecule or any other xenobiotic (**Figure 11**). The hydrophilicity of the drug molecule

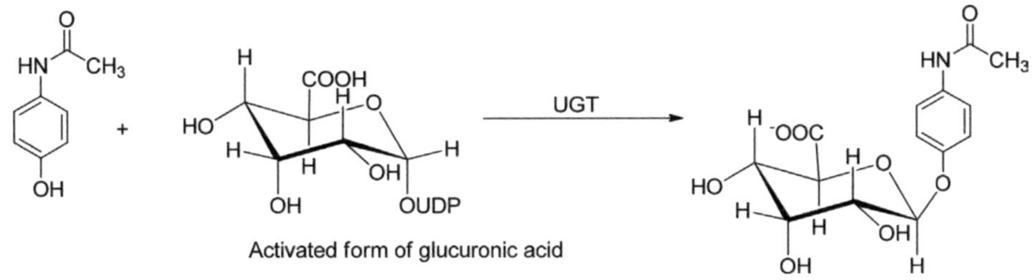

Figure 11.
Glucuronic acid conjugation of acetaminophen.

increases. Before attachment, it is converted into an activated form/moiety which is uridine diphosphate glucuronic acid (UDPGA). Uridine is a combination of uracil and ribose sugar. When uridine is attached to the phosphate group, then it is called uridine diphosphate [9].

This reaction occurs at (-OH, NH_2) hydrophilic site that is already introduced or unmarked during phase I reactions. The reaction is catalysed by uridine diphosphate glucuronosyltransferase (UGT) which is mainly present in liver and adjacent to CYP-450 in the endoplasmic reticulum (ER) of the liver. Drug molecules and activated form of glucuronic acid are present in the cytosol while UGT is present in SER so drug molecules and UDPGA are transferred to SER where glucuronic acid conjugation occurs and metabolite/conjugated product is transferred to the cytoplasm [10].

At physiological pH, the carboxylic (COOH) group of glucuronic acid becomes ionised. Then the whole conjugate molecule becomes ionised and this ionic form is excreted in the kidney by tubules. Some products of glucuronic acid conjugation are excreted into the bile. From the bile, they come into the intestine where enzyme glucuronidase is present which hydrolyses the conjugate and the active drug is reabsorbed from the small intestine into the systemic circulation and the process is called enterohepatic circulation [11].

The process of glucuronic acid conjugation usually terminates the pharmacological activity of drugs but in some cases drug is converted into an active form. For example, the conversion of morphine into morphine 6-glucuronide. Hydroxyl groups are attached at position 3 and 6 of morphine. When the conjugation occurs at position 6, a pharmacologically active metabolite is produced. Most of the drugs undergo glucuronic acid conjugation and it is the most important amongst phase II metabolic reactions. There is an abundant availability of glucose in the body. Glucuronic acid conjugation can also take place at amino group (-NH_2) group. Examples are sulfonamides and desipramine.

3.2 Sulfate conjugation (SO_4^-)

The process of sulfate conjugation takes place in drugs that contain hydrophilic groups such as hydroxyl and amino groups. Inorganic sulfate (SO_4^-) ion is a hydrophilic group. In the process of conjugation, the SO_4^- becomes attached to drug molecules/xenobiotics but first of all, sulfate is converted into an activated form called 3-phosphoadenosine-5-phosphosulfate (PAPS) (**Figure 12**). The activated form of SO_4^- reacts with the drug molecule. Sulfotransferases are enzymes which catalyse the transfer of sulfate from PAPS to the xenobiotic molecule [12].

DOI: http://dx.doi.org/10.5772/intechopen.112854

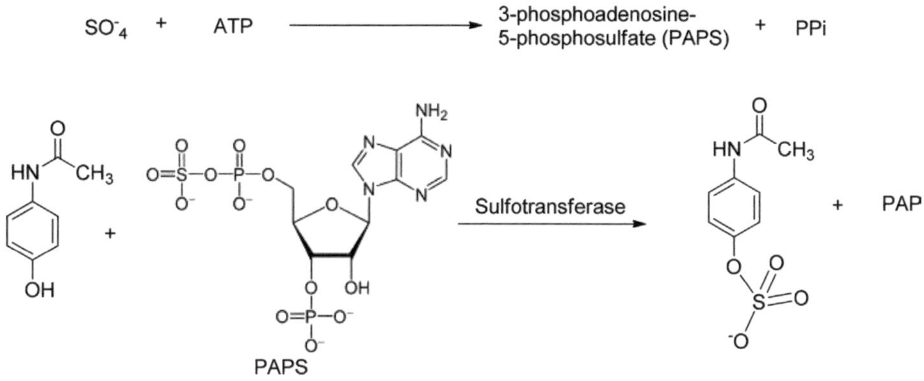

Figure 12.
Sulfate conjugation of acetaminophen.

Sulfate conjugation is catalysed by sulfotransferases and these enzymes are mostly present in the liver in the cytosol. Some sulfotransferases are also present in the Golgi apparatus. Sulfotransferases are also present in the intestine, brain and platelets of blood. Sulfate conjugation increases the hydrophilicity of drugs which are excreted from the body. Drugs which are metabolised by sulfate conjugation are endogenous steroids, catecholamines and other neurotransmitters. The pools of sulfate ions are limited in the body. Therefore, when a drug is administered for a longer time, then sulfate ions are depleted from the body. In this way, the process of glucuronic acid conjugation dominates [13].

3.3 Amino acid conjugation

The process of amino acid conjugation occurs in those drugs which contain carboxylic groups. For example, ibuprofen, ketoprofen and flurbiprofen. Glycine is the most important amino acid with which conjugation takes place but it also occurs with ornithine. In this reaction, there is the formation of a peptide bond between an amino acid and drug molecules. Amino acids are hydrophilic because they contain carboxylic and amino groups. First of all, drugs are converted into an activated form [14] (**Figure 13**). The carboxylic group of the drug reacts with ATP and the AMP ester of the drug is formed. Then co-enzyme A (CoSH) reacts with the AMP ester of the drug and the formation of the thioester is complete. In the third step, the amino acid glycine becomes attached to the drug molecule. The process of amino acid conjugation is catalysed by acyltransferase. The co-enzyme A regenerates at the end. Acyltransferase enzymes are located in the liver. By the attachment of glycine, the hydrophilicity of the drug increases and it is excreted from the body via kidney. Glycine conjugation also takes place at low doses but glucuronic acid conjugation dominates at large doses [3].

3.4 Glutathione conjugation

Glutathione (GSH) is a molecule which contains three amino acids i.e. Cysteine, glycine and glutamic acid. The process of glutathione conjugation takes place in drugs having electrophilic centres. These centres are created by electron-withdrawing groups. Some anticancer agents undergo the process of glutathione conjugation.

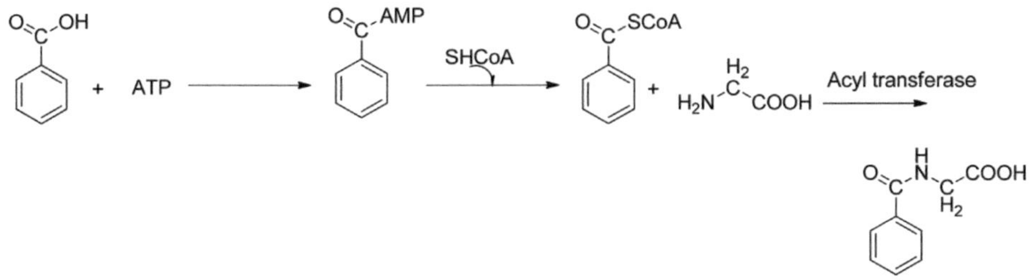

Figure 13.
Amino acid conjugation of xenobiotics.

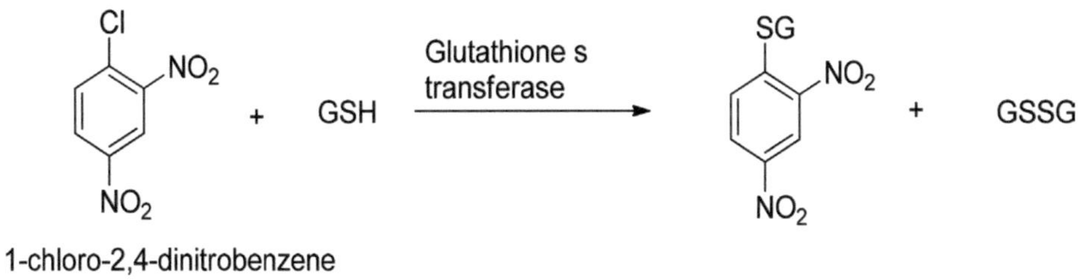

Figure 14.
Glutathione conjugation of a xenobiotic.

For example nitrogen mustards and nitrosoureas [15]. These drugs contain electron-withdrawing groups, they withdraw electrons, a positive charge is produced on the adjacent carbon atoms and it becomes electrophilic. Glutathione conjugation takes place between the drug and sulphhydryl group (SH) of glutathione (**Figure 14**). Glutathione ionises and hydrogen is removed from the SH group. A negative charge is developed on the sulphur atom. Glutathione conjugation does not require the activation of the endogenous molecule or substrate. This process is different from other conjugation reactions because glucuronic acid, sulfate and amino acid conjugations take place at nucleophilic centres. The glutathione conjugation is catalysed by glutathione-s-transferases located in the liver. Some glutathione conjugation reactions take place without the involvement of transferases. Most insecticides are metabolised by glutathione conjugation. Electron-withdrawing groups are also present in some insecticides and herbicides. Glutathione conjugation is the defensive mechanism of the body against toxic metabolites of foreign particles [16]. But glutathione is present in limited amounts in the body. If toxic compounds are ingested in large amount, the glutathione stores are depleted. In this situation, the body is exposed to the harmful effects of these metabolites. This conjugation reaction is a displacement or substitution reaction. When a drug is metabolised by glutathione conjugation it is not excreted from the body and it is further converted into mercapturic acid which is the end product. In this step, glutamic acid and glycine are cleaved from glutathione. Some scientists call it phase III metabolism [17].

3.5 Acetylation

The process of acetylation takes place in those drugs which contain amino group, hydrazine and hydrazide linkage in their structures. For example, sulfonamides and phenelzine etc. (**Figure 15**). In the process of acetylation, the amino group is

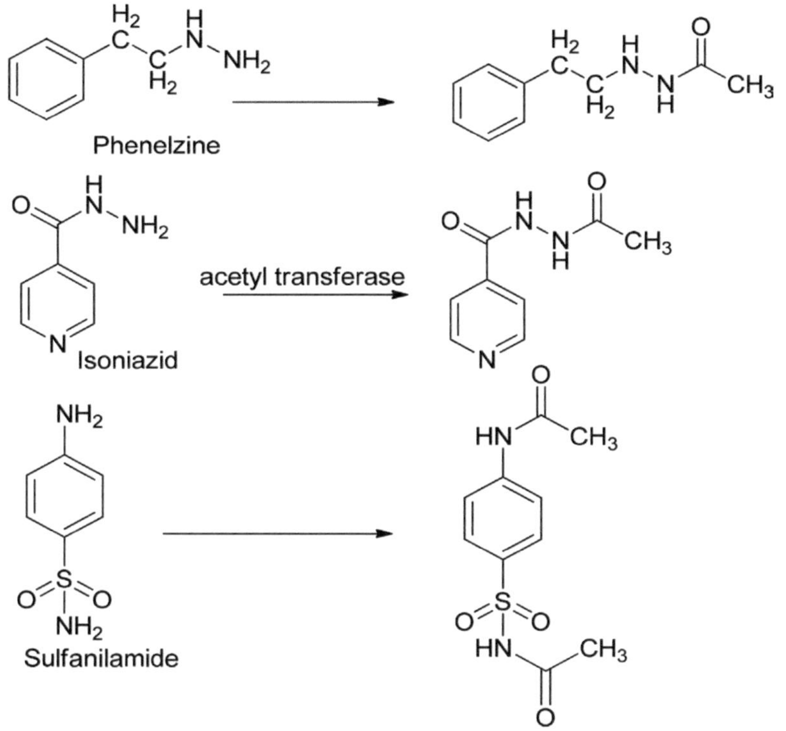

Figure 15.
Acetylation of drug molecules having amino group.

converted into an amide group. The acetyl group is provided by acetyl co-enzyme A. The acetyl co-enzyme A is formed by pyruvic acid, the end product of glycolysis [18]. Generally, phase II reaction increase the hydrophilicity of drugs but the acetylation does not increase hydrophilicity. The process of acetylation terminates the activity of drugs. Acetyltransferase is the enzyme that transfers the acetyl group from acetyl coenzyme-A to drugs. These enzymes are mainly present in the liver but also in RBCs and lungs. Populations are divided into fast acetylators and slow acetylators. Slow acetylators are exposed to the toxic effects of drugs [19].

3.6 Methylation

Methylation is a process in which methyl group becomes attached to the drug molecule. The process of methylation mostly takes place in endogenous molecules. For example neurotransmitters, noradrenaline is converted into adrenaline by methylation (**Figure 16**). In most cases, methylation results in the formation of biologically active molecules. But in some cases it produces inactive metabolites.

Methylation does not increase hydrophilicity because methyl group is lipophilic. Methyl group is provided by amino acid methionine. Methionine is converted into activated form which is called as S-adenosyl methionine. The process of methylation is catalysed by methyl transferases enzymes which are located in liver along with intestine and kidney [20]. There are three types of methylation i.e. N-methylation, O-methylation and S-methylation. Examples of N-methylation are conversion of noradrenaline into adrenaline, and histamine into n-methyl histamine. The conversion of

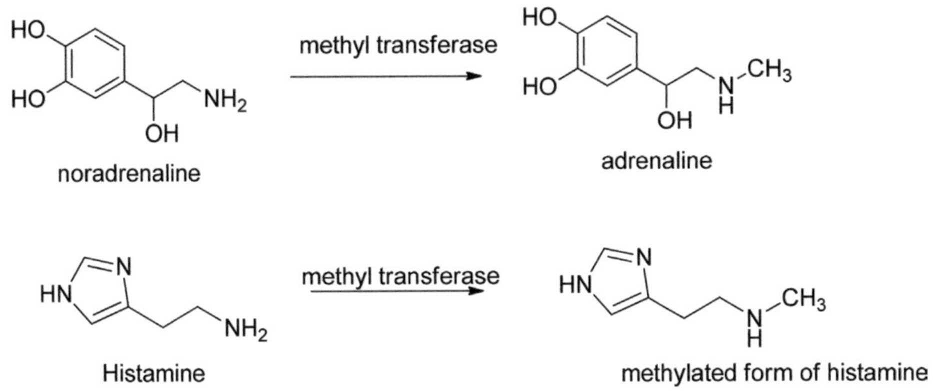

Figure 16.
Methylation of neurotransmitters.

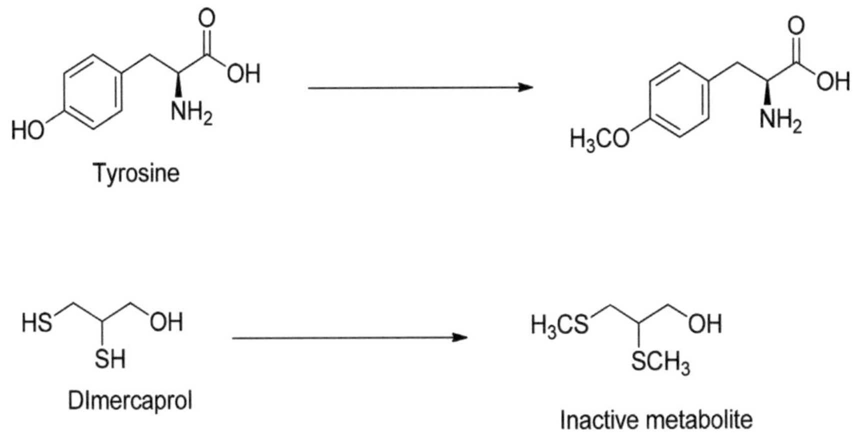

Figure 17.
Methylation of tyrosine and dimercaprol.

tyrosine into methoxy tyrosine and dimercaprol into methylated form are examples of O-methylation and S-methylation respectively (**Figure 17**). There are specific enzymes for each reaction.

4. Drug metabolism and drug design

The knowledge of drug metabolism is important in new drug design and development. If the new drug is quickly metabolised in the body, some non-reactive groups are added which resist the drug metabolism. For example, tolbutamide (**Figure 18**) is an anti-diabetic drug and it has a shorter half-life (2.5 hrs). It undergoes the process of metabolism and the methyl group converted into a carboxyl group. If the methyl group is replaced by the chlorine atom, then this compound (chlorpropamide) achieves a longer half-life (12–15 hrs) as compared to tolbutamide [21]. Drug metabolism has a significant effect on pharmacokinetic, pharmacodynamic and safety of a drug [22]. Some drugs are administered in inactive forms and are called as prodrugs. In prodrug, a drug is chemically modified to overcome its problems of absorption,

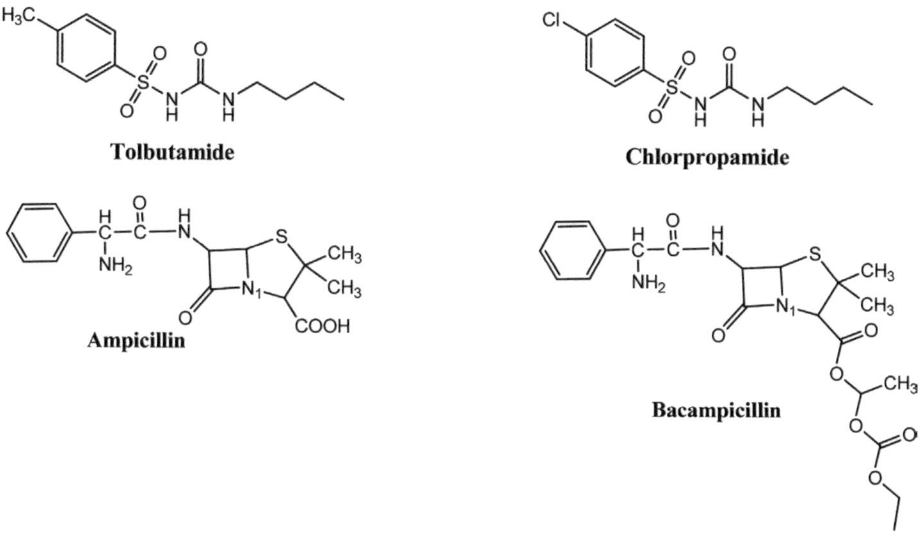

Figure 18.
Drug metabolism and drug design.

route of administration, metabolism and excretion. Prodrugs have labile functional groups which are easily metabolised in the body. For example, ester, phosphate, carbamate. Masking of polar functional improves oral bioavailability [23]. For example, chloramphenicol palmitate and bacampicillin are prodrugs of chloramphenicol and ampicillin respectively.

5. *In silico* pharmacokinetic studies

About 40% of new drugs fail in clinical trials because of poor pharmacokinetic properties. Nowadays pharmacokinetic properties of new compounds are evaluated by swissADME, ADMETlab and pkCSM web tools. 3D structure of compounds are generated on online software and pharmacokinetic properties ADMET (absorption, distribution, metabolism, excretion and toxicity) are computed. The GI absorption, BBB permeation, P-gp substrate, cytochrome P450 enzyme inhibition/induction, skin permeation are critical for the oral activity of drug molecules and these properties can be predicted. The prediction of pharmacokinetic properties helps to understand the behaviour of drug molecules in the human body. *In silico* predictions help to reduce the costly experimental approach [24]. The drug likeness of new molecules is also predicted by Lipinski rule of five [25]. According to this rule, drug molecules having more than five hydrogen bond donors, more than 10 hydrogen bond acceptor, logP more than five and molecular weight more 500 dalton are less likely to be orally active. High lipophilicity leads to the poor absorption of drug molecules. Similarly, compounds having big weights are less likely to absorb from GIT. About 80% drugs have molecular weight less than 450. The molecules having polar surface area less than 140°A and number of rotatable bond less than 10 also show good oral bioavailability. Drug molecules that follow the RO5 have increased chances of reaching the market and have less probability to fail during the clinical trials [26].

6. Conclusion

Drug metabolism is very significant in controlling the pharmacokinetics. Drug metabolising enzymes carry out the metabolism of endogenous as well as exogenous substances. Phase I metabolic reactions introduce a hydrophilic group in the drug molecules where phase II metabolic reactions can take place. In this chapter, we discussed the drug metabolic reactions and enzymes involved in these reactions. Most of the drugs are metabolised by CYP450 enzymes. The study of drug metabolism is essential for the safety and efficacy of drug molecules. The pharmacokinetic properties of drugs can be predicted by carrying out drug metabolism studies. The metabolic pathways of new drugs should be determined to predict the possibility of adverse drug reactions and drug-drug interactions.

Author details

Noor ul Amin Mohsin[1*], Maryam Farrukh[2], Saba Shahzadi[1] and Muhammad Irfan[3]

1 Faculty of Pharmaceutical Sciences, Department of Pharmaceutical Chemistry, Government College University Faisalabad, Pakistan

2 Faculty of Pharmaceutical Sciences, Department of Pharmacology, Government College University Faisalabad, Pakistan

3 Faculty of Pharmaceutical Sciences, Department of Pharmaceutics, Government College University Faisalabad, Pakistan

*Address all correspondence to: noorulaminmohsin@yahoo.com

References

[1] Nebert DW, Dalton TP. The role of cytochrome P450 enzymes in endogenous signalling pathways and environmental carcinogenesis. Nature Reviews Cancer. 2006;**6**(12):947-960

[2] Foye WO. Foye's Principles of Medicinal Chemistry. Philadelphia, USA: Lippincott Williams & Wilkins; 2008

[3] Lakshmanan M. Drug metabolism. In: Introduction to Basics of Pharmacology and Toxicology. Vol. 12019. Singapore: Springer; 2019. pp. 99-116

[4] Bortolussi S, Catucci G, Gilardi G, Sadeghi SJ. N-and S-oxygenation activity of truncated human flavin-containing monooxygenase 3 and its common polymorphic variants. Archives of Biochemistry Biophysics. 2021;**697**:108663

[5] Eh-Haj BM. Metabolic N-dealkylation and N-oxidation as elucidators of the role of alkylamino moieties in drugs acting at various receptors. Molecules. 2021;**26**(7):1917

[6] Marchitti SA, Brocker C, Stagos D, Vasiliou V. Non-P450 aldehyde oxidizing enzymes: The aldehyde dehydrogenase superfamily. Expert Opinion on Drug Metabolism Toxicology. 2008;**4**(6):697-720

[7] Guo Y, Lee H, Jeong H. Gut microbiota in reductive drug metabolism. Progress in Molecular Biology Translational Science. 2020;**171**:61-93

[8] Karaman R. Prodrugs design based on inter-and intramolecular chemical processes. Chemical Biology Drug Design. 2013;**82**(6):643-668

[9] Ionescu C, Caira MR. Drug Metabolism: Current Concepts. Dordrecht: Springer; 2005

[10] OuzzineM,GulbertiS,RamalanjaonaN, Magdalou J, Fournel-Gigleux S. The UDP-glucuronosyltransferases of the blood-brain barrier: Their role in drug metabolism and detoxication. Frontiers in Cellular Neuroscience. 2014;**8**:349

[11] Okour M, Brundage RC. Modeling enterohepatic circulation. Current Pharmacology Reports. 2017;**3**:301-313

[12] Järvinen E, Deng F, Kiander W, Sinokki A, Kidron H, Sjöstedt N. The role of uptake and efflux transporters in the disposition of glucuronide and sulfate conjugates. Frontiers in Pharmacology. 2022;**12**:802539

[13] Xie Y, Xie W. The role of sulfotransferases in liver diseases. Drug Metabolism Disposition. 2020;**48**(9):742-749

[14] Hou Y, Hu S, Li X, He W, Wu G. Amino acid metabolism in the liver: Nutritional and physiological significance. In: Amino Acids in Nutrition Health: Amino Acids in Systems Function Health. Cham: Springer; 2020. pp. 21-37

[15] Desideri E, Ciccarone F, Ciriolo MR. Targeting glutathione metabolism: Partner in crime in anticancer therapy. Nutrients. 2019;**11**(8):1926

[16] Hayes JD, Flanagan JU, Jowsey IR. Glutathione transferases. Annual Review of Pharmacology & Toxicology. 2005;**45**:51-88

[17] Hanna PE, Anders M. The mercapturic acid pathway. Critical Reviews in Toxicology. 2019;**49**(10):819-929

[18] Liu Y, Bai C. Engineered ethanol-driven biosynthetic system for improving

production of acetyl-CoA derived drugs in Crabtree-negative yeast. Metabolic Engineering. 2019;**54**:275-284

[19] Hein DW, Millner LM. Arylamine N-acetyltransferase acetylation polymorphisms: Paradigm for pharmacogenomic-guided therapy-A focused review. Expert Opinion on Drug Metabolism Toxicology. 2021;**17**(1):9-21

[20] Walvekar AS, Laxman S. Methionine at the heart of anabolism and signaling: Perspectives from budding yeast. Frontiers in Microbiology. 2019;**10**:2624

[21] Kumar GN, Surapaneni S. Role of drug metabolism in drug discovery and development. Medicinal Research Reviews. 2001;**21**(5):397-411

[22] Li Y, Meng Q, Yang M, et al. Current trends in drug metabolism and pharmacokinetics. Acta Pharmaceutica Sinica B. 2019;**9**(6):1113-1144

[23] Doss GA, Baillie TA. Addressing metabolic activation as an integral component of drug design. Drug Metabolism Reviews. 2006;**38**(4):641-649

[24] Alqahtani S. *In silico* ADME-Tox modeling: Progress and prospects. Expert Opinion on Drug Metabolism Toxicology. 2017;**13**(11):1147-1158

[25] Lipinski CA. Lead-and drug-like compounds: The rule-of-five revolution. Drug Discovery Today: Technologies. 2004;**1**(4):337-341

[26] Leeson PD, Springthorpe B. The influence of drug-like concepts on decision-making in medicinal chemistry. Nature Reviews Drug Discovery. 2007;**6**(11):881-890

Chapter 3

Drug Induced Hematological Disorders: An Undiscussed Stigma

Sharad Chand, Manoj S. Dikkatwar, Ramesh Datta Pant, Vinamra Misra, Niharika Pradhan, Urooj Ansari and Gourab Debnath

Abstract

Drug Induced Hematological Disorders (DIHD) are one among the most frequently encountered Adverse Drug Reactions (ADRs) among the patients using the systemic drug therapy. These unwanted and noxious incidents are often unnoticed or even neglected most of the time during the clinical practices. However, they largely affect the compliance of the patients with their therapy and subsequently affecting the therapeutic outcome of the drug regimen. The inception of the concept of Pharmacovigilance has largely enlightened on this neglected issue and raised the concern over several scientific sessions. However, this serious issue remained unaddressed clinically. These noxious conditions frequently provoke the adverse events or precipitate the underlying medical complications affecting the safety of the patients. The wise and vigilant use of certain risky medication capable of inducing such clinical conditions can significantly reduce these incidences. Thus, the utilization of the skills and the expertise knowledge of the clinical pharmacist can play a pivotal role in preventing and minimizing such events.

Keywords: blood, drug induced disorders, adverse drug reactions, pharmacovigilance, clinical pharmacist, patient safety

1. Introduction

Drugs are now become part of our day-to-day life. The burden of disease in the ever-rising trend and the medical fraternity is progressing exponentially. The pharmaceutical industries are constantly expanding the spectrum of the pharmaceutical by carrying out the research and discovering the newer drugs or by synthesizing the molecule with the better efficacy. All the newer molecule or the formulations released in the market go through the strict regulatory process of their testing for safety and efficacy in the clinical subjects. However, it is not possible to the study the drugs completely. Thus, none of the drugs available in the markets are completely safe [1].

The molecule goes through the laboratory studies followed by the pre-clinical and clinical studies and the molecule able to demonstrate the sufficient safety along with the promising efficacy only will release in the market. This procedure generally takes the longtime of decade or even two-three decades [2]. Study of any marketed product after their release in the market is known as the post-marketing surveillance. Several of drugs with potentiality to threat the safety of the patients are continuously studied during this phase and the drugs with the established causality relationship with the adverse events are then recalled by the regulatory or the safety agencies. The Indian Pharmacopeial commission is one of the apex bodies to continuously monitor the safety of the drugs and collects the signals of the suspected adverse drug reactions [3].

Drug induced disorders are technically the adverse drug reactions occurred by that drug molecule or by the excipients used in the formulation of the drugs. The drug induces the adverse drug reactions by either pharmacokinetic or by the pharmacodynamic mechanism. Some of the most commonly occurring adverse drug reactions are drug induced liver disorders, drug induced pulmonary disorders, drug induced hematological disorders, drug induced renal disorders or any dermatological manifestations [4, 5]. Whatever may be the reactions, this incident possesses great risk to the patient safety and accounts for several injuries and casualties. These unwanted and noxious events generally remain undiagnosed or under-reported due to the various factors. However, the medical sciences are becoming vigilant toward such bitter event and continuously trying to detect, assess, manage, document, and prevent them [6–8].

Drug-induced hematological disorders (DIHD) are one among the major type of adverse drug reactions (ADRs) due to their severity rather than their incidence rate. The incidence rate of the DIHD is less compared to other ADRs, however, they posses the greater risk of morbidity and mortality. Thus, they are rare phenomenon occurring in the clinical setting. Some of the most frequently occurring DIHDs are Drug induced aplastic anemia, followed by drug induced agranulocytosis, megaloblastic and hemolytic anemia. There are few literatures in the scientific databases even reporting the incidences of drug induced thrombocytopenia. The incidence of these event is rare and the majority of ADRs are occurring after the chronic use of the medications. Thus, these ADRs are difficult to identify during the clinical trials and are best detected during the post-marketing surveillance [9–11].

2. Types of drug-induced hematological disorders

There are several types of hematological disorders occurring as an adverse drug reaction of drugs, most common types of them are [12, 13]:

1. Drug-induced aplastic Anemia,

2. Drug-induced agranulocytosis

3. Drug-induced megaloblastic anemia

4. Drug-induced thrombocytopenia

5. Drug-induced hemolytic anemia [14–17].

2.1 Drug-induced aplastic anemia

This is the clinical condition characterized by extremely low count of blood cells due to the inability of the bone marrow to produce the sufficient amount of new blood cells [18–21]. This is an extremely condition and is generally life-threatening reactions associated with some category of drugs. These drugs are generally having their toxic effect toward the bone marrow and affect the process of blood cell synthesis. This is again life-threatening condition due to its impact on all types of blood cells including white blood cells (WBC), red blood corpuscles (RBC) and platelets (Thrombocyte). Thus, the condition is clinically interpreted by the decline in all types of blood cells.

2.1.1 Mechanism involved or pathophysiology of the drug-induced aplastic anemia

The underlying mechanism to induce the aplastic anemia is the activation of the immune complex by these suspected drugs and the patient's own immune system is directed toward the bone marrow. The immune related injury to the bone marrow will results in the synthesis of limited number of blood cells (hypoplastic anemia) or sometime make them almost empty (aplastic anemia).

Another hypothesis states that there is the generation of the intermediate toxic compounds that binds to several functional proteins and deoxyribose-nuclease acid (DNA) of these hematopoietic bone marrow cells leading to the direct injury of bone marrow. However, the generation of these toxic intermediate is highly dependent to the genetic variability of an individual. Some of the other research suggests the generation of toxic intermediates as an idiosyncratic condition.

2.1.2 List of common drugs responsible for aplastic anemia

- *Salicylates:* Aspirin
- *Antimalarial:* Chloroquine
- *Diuretics:* Hydrochlorothiazide, furosemide, thiazide
- *Antibiotics:* Chloramphenicol, sulphonamides, penicillamines
- *Anti-neoplastic agents:* Propylthiouracil
- *Anticonvulsants:* Carbamazepine, phenytoin
- *Miscellaneous:* Benzene containing compounds, drugs containing heavy metals.

2.1.3 Clinical manifestations of drug-induced aplastic anemia

The most significant clinical presentation of aplastic anemia is the decline in the count of blood cells and the condition is widely termed as pancytopenia. Aplastic anemia can be clinical characterized by either decrease in one type of blood cells or by the overall decrease of blood cells in most of the cases. Some of the other clinical features are:

- White blood cells fall below 3500cells/mm^3
- Hemoglobin level fall below 10gm%
- Complain of easy tiredness and fatigue by the patients

- Generalized weakness and feeling of drainage of energy
- Thrombocyte counts fall below 55,000 cells/mm^3
- Incident of prolonged bleedings
- Epistaxis
- Gum bleeding
- Fever (Mild to moderate)
- High propensity for acquiring the infections
- Reticulocyte count fall below 30,000 cells/mm^3
- There might be the fall of the blood cells counts signifying the severity of the aplastic anemia and the fall of reticulocyte index to 1%, neutrophil level to 500 cells/ mm^3 and platelet levels to 20,000 cells/mm^3 is the indication of severe aplastic anemia.
- The condition of aplastic anemia can be life threatening if its level goes beyond the levels of severe aplastic anemia.

2.2 Drug-induced agranulocytosis

This is a clinical condition where there is a decrease in the body's total number of mature myeloid cells (Granulocytes and immature ones) to 500 cells/mm^3 or fewer [22–25]. Occurrence of agranulocytosis is mainly seen in females and aged people with an approximated yearly incidence rate of one to 12 cases per 10 lacs population. This hematological condition will generally settle over time with approving care and prevention and management of infection.

2.2.1 Mechanism involved or pathophysiology of the drug-induced agranulocytosis (DIA)

The exact reason for drug induced agranulocytosis is still not recognized but many mechanisms were put forward, nonetheless the recent studies revealed that medications may have a direct toxic effect on the bone marrow, neutrocytes or stem cells. The first mechanism involves the anti-thyroid drugs (ATD) such as methimazole and propylthiouracil which have been outlined to cause agranulocytosis. Apoptosis occur which activates inflammasomes (important for innate immune system). The following figure shows the direct toxicity of ATD-Induced agranulocytosis. In recent outline 7–23% of DIA cases occur due to anti-thyroid drugs. Higher dose of methimazole received by patient showed neutropenia.

The second kind of mechanism comprises antibodies, neutrophils, immune-mediated medications, or drug metabolites. This process suggests that the medication is adsorbing through the neutrophile membrane. The drug-containing membrane functions as a hapten to promote the production of antibodies. As a result of the antibodies' binding to the drug-membrane complex, the phagocytic system activates

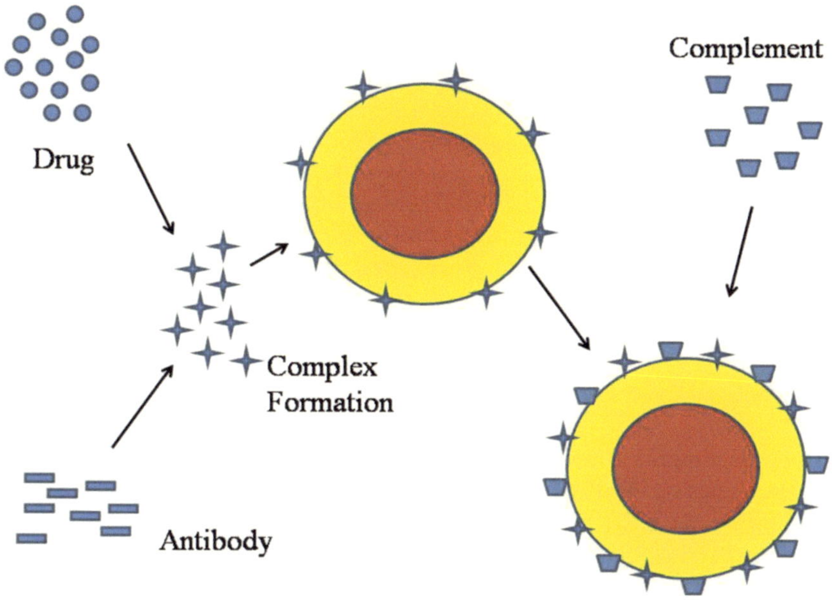

Figure 1.
Antibody and complement system-based mechanism of toxicity.

complement, which in turn causes the WBC to be destroyed. When medications like penicillin derivatives are administered at larger doses, this hapten-type response occurs as depicted in **Figure 1**.

There are also several other immune-mediated processes that have been identified. The culprit medicine reforms the neutrophil membrane through the autoantibodies forming to a membrane mechanism. This alteration triggers the production of autoantibodies, which kill cells.

2.2.2 List of common drugs responsible for agranulocytosis

Anti-thyroid drug (ATD): Carbimazole, methimazole, propylthiouracil.
Beta-lactam antibiotics: penicillin, penicillamine, ampicillin.
Anticonvulsants: Carbamazepine.
Cardiac glycosides: Digoxin, digitalis.
Propranolol: beta blockers.
Corticosteroids: Prednisone.
ACE-inhibitors: Captopril.
Anti-infectives: Dapsone.

2.2.3 Clinical features of drug-induced agranulocytosis

Symptoms of agranulocytosis occurs rapidly in less than a weeks after the intake of culprit drug.

- Having a sore throat is a very common symptom
- Complains of discomfort, illness

- People being febrile
- Increased propensity toward infections

2.3 Drug-induced megaloblastic anemia

A condition where the growth of RBC precursors (Megaloblasts) in the bone marrow is aberrant [26–28]. Drugs including amino salicylic acid, colchicine, neomycin, and metformin can prevent the absorption of vitamin B12. Megaloblastic anemia from these agents is extremely uncommon because of how little B12 the body needs and how much of it is present in most diets.

2.3.1 Pathophysiology of drug induced megaloblastic anemia

Megaloblastic anemia is most frequently brought on by cobalamin (vitamin B12) or folate insufficiency (vitamin B9). For the development of healthy cells, such as the precursors of red blood cells, these two vitamins act as building blocks. Since most dietary causes of folate and vitamin B12 deficiency may be resolved, drugs have emerged as a more significant contributor to megaloblastic anemia. Megaloblasts-inducing medications are frequently employed in clinical settings, although the caused changes to DNA synthesis pathways aren't always welcomed. The most crucial biochemical process during DNA synthesis is the synthesis of thymidine, which is a component of DNA but not RNA. As a result, it is susceptible to drug inhibition. Through the methylation of pyrimidine, which is a folate and vitamin B12 dependent process, thymidine is produced. Megaloblastosis is brought on by medications that physically destroy vitamins, compete with reducing enzymes, or obstruct folate or vitamin B12 absorption, transport, or delivery.

2.3.2 Causative drugs

- *Anticonvulsants*: Phenytoin
- *Barbiturates*: Phenobarbital
- *Anticonvulsants*: Primidone
- *Antimetabolites*: Methotrexate
- *Sulphonamides*: Cotrimoxazole
- *Biguanides*: Metformin
- *Nucleoside reverse transcriptase inhibitors (NRTIs)*: Zidovudine
- *Antimetabolites*: 5-Flurouracil

2.3.3 Clinical manifestation

- Shortness of Breath
- Malaise

- Muscle Weakness
- Irregular Heartbeats
- Dizziness

2.4 Drug-induced thrombocytopenia

A disorder known as thrombocytopenia occurs when there are not enough platelets in the blood [29–31]. Blood cells called platelets aid in blood clotting. Bleeding risk is increased by a low platelet count. When thrombocytopenia is present, the platelet count falls below 104 cells/mm^3 or falls below 50% of the normal level. About 10 cases/105 people are affected by drug-induced thrombocytopenia per year. Except for cases linked to heparin, none of the numerous epidemiological studies have been reported. Find patient-specific risk factors for medication-induced thrombocytopenia that do not just involve exposure to drug classes.

2.4.1 Mechanism involved or pathophysiology of the drug-induced thrombocytopenia anemia

DITP is a distinctive immune-mediated reaction. Medication-dependent antibodies are a rare family of antibodies that bind securely to platelet surface glycoprotein epitopes only when a sensitizing drug is present. Drug-dependent antibodies are very sensitive to the chemical makeup of drugs. According to this hypothesis, medicines bind non-covalently and reversibly to antibodies as well as platelets, generally at locations on GP IIb-IIIa and/or GP Ib-V-IX. The resulting "sandwich" (seen in **Figure 2**) encourages the development of strong interactions between the antibody and platelet epitopes. The Fab domains' capacity to identify medicines bound to platelet epitopes is used to select the antibodies that are produced because of exposure to sensitizers. Antiplatelet antibodies that are dependent on a medicine typically start to show up 1 to 2 weeks after first exposure. Drug-dependent antibodies may also develop following prolonged, irregular drug use. Unlike neutrophils and erythrocytes, platelets are significantly more frequently the target of drug-dependent antibodies for unexplained reasons.

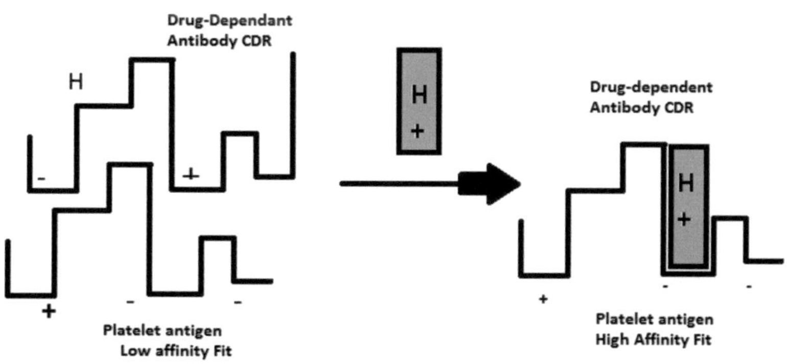

Figure 2.
Drug-dependent model with specific affinity with thrombocytes.

2.4.2 Clinical features of drug-induced thrombocytopenia

The most significant clinical feature of thrombocytopenia is significant drop in the platelet count (<50% of normal platelet range). Due to the platelet count drop lots of sign and symptoms may noticed in patients like,

- In this case platelet count in the blood drops below 10,0000 cells/mm^3
- Abnormal bleeding.
- Bleeding when brushing teeth.
- Easy bruising
- Red spots (petechiae) on the skin.

2.5 Drug-induced Hemolytic Anemia

Haemolytic anemia is a blood condition that occurs primarily when red blood cells are destroyed faster than they can be replaced [32–34]. Red blood cells are normally released from the bone marrow and survive for about 120 days before being cleared by phagocytic cells in the spleen and liver. The process by which immature red blood cells are destroyed is called haemolysis. This haemolysis occurs due to red blood cell defects or abnormal changes in the intravascular environment. Both processes may facilitate drug-induced haemolysis. It can develop rapidly or slowly and can be mild or severe.

2.5.1 Mechanism involved or pathophysiology of drug induced hemolytic anemia

Drug-induced haemolytic anemia is a type of blood disorder in which the body's defense system is triggered by drugs, resulting in an attack on its own red blood cells. This leads to premature destruction of red blood cells, known as haemolysis. The drug causes the immune system to see its own red blood cells as foreign. The body responds by producing antibodies that destroy its own red blood cells. Immunoglobulin G (IgG) and/or immunoglobulin M (IgM) bind to antigens on the surface of red blood cells and begin to destroy them.

2.5.2 List of common drugs responsible for hemolytic anemia

- *Antibiotics:* Cephalosporins, Beta-lactum antibiotics, Ciprofloxacin
- *Diuretics:* Hydrochlorothiazide
- *Antihypertensives:* Methyldopa,
- *Antiarrhythmic:* Qiunidine, Procainamide
- *NSAIDS:* Diclofenac,
- *Insulin secretagogues:* Sulfonylureas

- *Proton-pump inhibitors:* Omeprazole, lansoprazole
- *Miscellaneous:* Acetaminophen, levodopa, probenecid, erythromycin

2.5.3 Clinical features of drug-induced immune hemolytic anemia

The sign and symptoms resemble the clinical features like anemia, patient may complain of fever with chills and rigor, breathlessness etc.

2.6 Identification of drug-induced hematological disorders

The adverse event of drug induced hematological disorders are best identified during the clinical use of the suspected drugs. The patients administrating the suspected drug with potential to induce these hematological events should be closely monitored and any suspicious events should be assessed for the causal relationship with the drugs using the causality assessment scale. There are several scales to establish the causal relationship, assess the severity and preventability of the drugs with these adverse effects. The suspected drug should be withdrawn immediately, and the drug should not be rechallenged as these incidences are severe in nature. The suspected adverse drug reactions are then submitted to the local, zonal, or regional pharmacovigilance centers. The reporting can also be done to the competent authorities by their website with the complete information of the events and product.

2.7 Diagnosis tools

2.7.1 History taking

The complete and detailed history taking helps in diagnosing most of the cases. The patients usually have the history of taking the medications susceptible to induce these adverse drug reactions.

2.7.2 Monitoring of therapy

The monitoring of the therapy containing these agents also help in the prevention or early detection of such events.

2.7.3 Laboratory findings

The other mean to diagnose the cases are to obtaining the laboratory report and clinical correlation to the past medication history. The laboratory reports show the decline in the blood cells post commencement of medication therapy. Laboratory tests mainly performed are:

2.7.3.1 Complete blood count (CBC)

This test measures the levels of platelets and other blood cells in the blood.

2.7.3.2 Blood smear

A portion of patients' blood is placed on a glass slide under the microscope to observe the platelets.

2.7.4 Bone marrow examination

These tests check to see if the bone marrow is healthy.

2.7.5 Vigilant use of risky medication

Some drugs with the frequent occurrence of aplastic anemia are chloramphenicol and propyl thiouracil thus, these therapy needs to be monitored.

2.7.6 Study of factors affecting the ADRs

There are various intra and intersubjective variability including the immunological factors, genetic factors, pharmacokinetics, and pharmacodynamics factors. Such factors can be identified and documented for some vulnerable patients. Early diagnosis is important to limit the injury caused by the drugs and restore the peripheral count of blood cells.

2.8 Management

2.8.1 Goals of therapy of DIHD

- The mains' goal of drug induced hematological disorder is to ameliorate the ADR by timely withdrawal of suspected medications.

- Timely assessment and identification of any insult to the hematopoietic system caused by any suspected drugs.

- Another goal is to ensure the safe therapy and warn the patients about the drugs and their probable ADRs in future.

- To limit the decline in the blood cells.

- To minimize the risk of infection and bleeding.

2.8.2 Specific treatment of drug-induced aplastic anemia

- Immediate withdrawal of the culprit drugs. The removal of the culprit drug will arrest the insult to the hematopoietic system and reverse the condition.

- Fever can be treated by use of antipyretics and broad-spectrum antibiotics. However, the recent evidence suggests that the patients should not be administered with broad spectrum antibiotics as a chemoprophylaxis.

- Treating the adverse drug reactions by administering another drug is not recommendable.

- Generally mild aplastic anemia will reverse over the time and no specific treatment is required. The nature of specific treatment depends upon the level of cytopenia. The extreme low level of blood cells needs to be replaced by the transfusion as per clinical need.

- Immunosuppressive therapy and use of corticosteroids (methylprednisolone and/or prednisolone 1 mg/kg/day up to months or 6 weeks) can be warranted in the typical case of drug induced aplastic anemia due to the involvement of immunological system. E.g., antithymocyte globulin and cyclosporine.

- Hemopoietic stem cell transplantation can be suggested in the extreme cases. But rejection of therapy is the major challenge in this approach.

2.8.3 Specific treatment of drug-induced agranulocytosis

- Immediate withdrawal of the culprit drug.

- Filgrastim and sargramostim lessen the timeline of neutropenia, and the line antibiotic therapy, with hospital stay.

- Fever can be treated by use of antipyretics and broad-spectrum antibiotics.

- Treating the adverse drug reactions by administering another drug is not recommendable.

2.8.4 Specific treatment of drug-induced megaloblastic anemia

- Most individuals are treated with cobalamin or folate once drug-induced megaloblastic alterations and myelodysplasia-related megaloblasts have been ruled out. Due to the progressive development of megaloblastic anaemias, many patients can cope with low hemoglobin levels and do not need blood transfusions. Only individuals with severe, uncomplicated, and life-threatening anemia should get transfusion therapy.

- The causative agents of megaloblastosis must be identified to manage and treat drug-induced megaloblastic anemia. If there is an alternative, it will take the place of the cause. However, if the chemotherapeutic treatment that caused the anemia were to be stopped, there would be no real therapeutic alternative, and the anemia would then become a tolerable side effect. In this situation, ensuring appropriate consumption of folate and vitamin B12 is necessary. Additionally, when medical professionals utilize substances that prevent DNA synthesis, they should exercise additional caution. Folate antagonists and purine and pyrimidine analogues are stronger and can cause anemia very quickly. As a result, it is advised to employ less strong inhibitors; however, megaloblastic anemia may progress more slowly in this situation.

- There is no effective treatment for chemotherapy-related drug-induced megaloblastic anemia, hence the condition is tolerated as a side effect of treatment. If cotrimoxazole causes drug induced megaloblastic anemia, a trial course of folic acid, 5 to 10 mg up to four times per day, can treat the anemia. The megaloblastic anemia brought on by either phenytoin or phenobarbital is frequently treated with folic acid supplementation of 1 mg per day, but some practitioners contend that this can lessen the efficiency of the antiepileptic drugs.

2.8.5 Specific treatment of drug induced thrombocytopenia

- Immediate withdrawal of the culprit drug.
- Platelet interfering drugs should be avoided like Heparin, Clopidogrel etc.
- Corticosteroids or IV immunoglobulin may be given for suspected immune thrombocytopenia.
- If the patient's thrombocytopenia condition in severe and bleeding in there, platelet transfusion can be given.

2.8.6 Specific treatment hemolytic anemia

- Immediate withdrawal of the culprit drugs. The removal of the culprit drug will stop the destruction it may be causing to red blood cells and reverse the condition.
- Glucocorticoids containing drug may find their clinical implications in the serious cases.
- Additional treatment contains the use of monoclonal antibodies like anti-CD20, rituximab and other modified immunoglobulins. However, they always possess the serious ADRs.

2.9 Prevention of drug induced hematological disorders

- Drug induced hematological disorders are often unpredictable, rare and life-threatening adverse drug reactions. These incidences can be minimized by adopting the following preventive measures.
- Obtain the detailed medical and medication history.
- Make a note of previous drug-allergy.
- Avoid designing the complex therapy by adding the multiple drugs as the polypharmacy is one among the major reason for ADRs.
- Patient should avoid taking the medication from the pharmacy store without any proper prescription.
- The patient prescribed with the potential drug needs to be counseled for the expected side effects and ADRs and educate them to report to the hospital immediately after occurrence of such events.
- Utilizing the specialist service of clinical pharmacist in educating the patients, creating awareness, drug therapy review and optimization of drug and individualizing the drug therapy can prevent the occurrence of these event.
- Timely prediction, assessment, and management of these event can prevent the magnitude of injury and helps in the prevention of occurrence.

- The patients with the known drug sensitivity can be alerted by providing the yellow card.

- Monitoring of the therapy for the prescribed time to find any unwanted events.

3. Conclusions

Drug use became a part of healthcare delivery system in the modern days. The marketed drugs pass the stringent approval process from the regulatory authorities. However, they carry the possible threat of serious adverse effects among the patients. All the drugs are associated with side effects ranging from mild to life threatening effect. The drug induced blood disorders are one among the major class of adverse drug reactions. The vigilant use of these medications may help in early detection and management of this drug induced events. These events are preventable in large scale by adopting the safe health care delivery system by adopting the expert knowledges in the multi-disciplinary team. The drug induced events are unavoidable, but the incidences can be prevented, or the severity can be flattened in majority of cases.

Author details

Sharad Chand[1*], Manoj S. Dikkatwar[1], Ramesh Datta Pant[2], Vinamra Misra[1], Niharika Pradhan[1], Urooj Ansari[1] and Gourab Debnath[1]

1 Department of Pharmacy Practice, Amity Institute of Pharmacy, Amity University Uttar Pradesh, Noida, India

2 LabCorp Drug Development India Private Limited, Bangalore, India

*Address all correspondence to: sureechand193@gmail.com

References

[1] Berdigaliyev N, Aljofan M. An overview of drug discovery and development. Future Medicinal Chemistry. 2020;**12**(10):939-947

[2] Umscheid CA, Margolis DJ, Grossman CE. Key concepts of clinical trials: A narrative review. Postgraduate Medicine. 2011;**123**(5):194-204

[3] Schultz A, Saville BR, Marsh JA, Snelling TL. An introduction to clinical trial design. Paediatric Respiratory Reviews. 2019;**32**:30-35

[4] Chand S, Bhandari R, Girish HN, Sukeerthi D, Sah SK, Voora L. Isoniazid induced psychosis. Journal of Global Pharma Technology. 2019;**11**(5):11-14

[5] Garratty G. Drug-induced immune cytopenia. Transfusion Medicine Reviews. 1993;**7**(4):213-214

[6] Voora L, Shastry CS, Bhandari R, Sukeerthi D, Rawal KB, Chand S. Phenytoin-induced erythroderma. Journal of Young Pharmacists. 2019;**11**(3):320-321

[7] Rachana J, Shastry CS, Mateti UV, Sharma R, Nandakumar UP, Chand S. Incidence and associated factors of adverse drug reactions in the general medicine department of a tertiary care teaching hospital. International Journal of Pharmaceutical Research. 2019;**11**(3):177-184

[8] Ammus S, Yunis AA. Drug-induced red cell dyscrasias. Blood Reviews. 1989;**3**(2):71-82

[9] Roy DA, Shanfar I, Shenoy P, Chand S, et al. Drug-related problems among chronic kidney disease patients: A pharmacist-led study. International Journal of Pharmaceutical Research. 2020;**12**(04):79-84

[10] Weil PG. Drug-induced blood dyscrasias. Canadian Medical Association Journal. 1962;**87**(13):685-689

[11] Sanija P, Nandakumar UP, Shetty J, Bharathraj KC, Vinay BC, Chand S, et al. Adverse drug reactions and its management associated with cancer chemotherapy. International Journal of Research in Pharmaceutical Sciences. 2020;**11**(04):5828-5835

[12] Iwase Y, Tsutsui N. Drug-induced blood toxicity. Nihon Yakurigaku Zasshi. 2008;**132**(6):343-346

[13] Dipiro JT. Pharmacotherapy: A pathophysiologic approach. 8th ed. New York: McGraw Hill education

[14] Danielson DA, Douglas SW 3rd, Herzog P, Jick H, Porter JB. Drug-induced blood disorders. Journal of the American Medical Association. 1984;**252**(23):3257-3260

[15] Nishimura J, Motomura S, Akagi T. Drug-induced hematological disorders. Nihon Rinsho. 2007;**65**(Suppl 8):99-105

[16] Shander A, Javidroozi M, Ashton ME. Drug-induced anemia and other red cell disorders: A guide in the age of polypharmacy. Current Clinical Pharmacology. 2011;**6**(4):295-303

[17] Huhn D. Medikamentös induzierte Störungen der Hämatopoese [drug-induced disorders of hematopoiesis]. Deutsche Medizinische Wochenschrift. 1980;**105**(45):1576-1581

[18] Malkin D, Koren G, Saunders EF. Drug-induced aplastic anemia:

Pathogenesis and clinical aspects. The American Journal of Pediatric Hematology/Oncology. 1990;**12**(4):402-410

[19] Pisciotta AV. Drug-induced leukopenia and aplastic anemia. Clinical Pharmacology and Therapeutics. 1971;**12**(1):13-43

[20] Nagai J, Matsukawa T, Suto K, Oshimi K, Miyagishima T. Aplastic anemia following drug-induced liver injury. Rinshō Ketsueki. 2019;**60**(7):779-784

[21] Thomas D, Moisidis A, Tsiakalos A, Alexandraki K, Syriou V, Kaltsas G. Antithyroid drug-induced aplastic anemia. Thyroid. 2008;**18**(10):1043-1048

[22] Lhomme F, Ochmann M, Lamy T. Agranulocytose Médicamenteuse [drug-induced agranulocytosis]. La Revue du Praticien. 2015;**65**(5):697-700

[23] Garbe E. Non-chemotherapy drug-induced agranulocytosis. Expert Opinion on Drug Safety. 2007;**6**(3):323-335

[24] Vicente N, Cardoso L, Barros L, Carrilho F. Antithyroid drug-induced agranulocytosis: State of the art on diagnosis and management. Drugs R D. 2017;**17**(1):91-96

[25] Pick AM, Nystrom KK. Nonchemotherapy drug-induced neutropenia and agranulocytosis: Could medications be the culprit? Journal of Pharmacy Practice. 2014;**27**(5):447-452

[26] Hesdorffer CS, Longo DL. Drug-induced megaloblastic Anemia. The New England Journal of Medicine. 2015;**373**(17):1649-1658

[27] Ben Salem C, Sakhri J, Hmouda H. Drug-induced megaloblastic Anemia. The New England Journal of Medicine. 2016;**374**(7):696

[28] Hesdorffer CS, Longo DL. Drug-induced megaloblastic Anemia. The New England Journal of Medicine. 2016;**374**(7):696-697

[29] Danese E, Montagnana M, Favaloro EJ, Lippi G. Drug-induced thrombocytopenia: Mechanisms and laboratory diagnostics. Seminars in Thrombosis and Hemostasis. 2020;**46**(3):264-274

[30] Kam T, Alexander M. Drug-induced immune thrombocytopenia. Journal of Pharmacy Practice. 2014;**27**(5):430-439

[31] Bakchoul T, Marini I. Drug-associated thrombocytopenia. Hematology. American Society of Hematology. Education Program. 2018;**2018**(1):576-583

[32] Renard D, Rosselet A. Drug-induced hemolytic anemia: Pharmacological aspects. Transfusion Clinique et Biologique. 2017;**24**(3):110-114

[33] Gehrs BC, Friedberg RC. Autoimmune hemolytic anemia. American Journal of Hematology. 2002;**69**(4):258-271

[34] Terada H. Drug-induced hemolytic anemia. Nihon Rinsho. 2007;**65**(Suppl. 8): 473-477

Section 2

Metabolomics and Drug Discovery

Chapter 4

Metabolomics: Special Emphasis on Basic Drug Discovery and Development

Dipankar Nath and Dipak Chetia

Abstract

Metabolomics utilizes analytical profiling technique for measuring and comparing large numbers of metabolites produced in the biological fluids. Traditional process of drug development is not sufficient enough to understand the proper biochemical processes within the targets which may finally lead to the failure. Metabolomics can be very useful to overcome such failure as it involves in the detailed profiling and understanding of the biochemical processes which helps in identification of target engagement (TE) markers as well as predicting mode of action (MOA). Currently pharmaceutical companies are utilizing this approach in the early drug development stage to combat failure. This chapter will mainly highlight the advantages of this concept over traditional concept of drug development along with recent developments of it.

Keywords: metabolomics, drug, disease, drug discovery and development, analytical approaches

1. Introduction

Pharmaceutical company that wants to thrive in this highly competitive field of introducing novel therapeutic agents for a variety of ailments at an extremely high pace, must devote a significant number of resources to the process of drug discovery. To create newer, more potent, and safer medications, they must make strides and look at different possibilities. The drug development process scenario has seen significant change since the turn of the twenty-first century [1].

From the initial step of target validation through clinical trials to clinical practice, the drug development process is a drawn-out, painful, and incredibly expensive one. The net output of such a method has also been subpar and frequently results from small improvements in currently available therapeutic agents. The current paradigm for drug development asks for the discovery of particular molecular targets that can be used to create highly powerful and selective inhibitors with little off-target activity. These substances may be synthetic small compounds that need medicinal chemistry optimization, or they may be natural products and their synthetic derivatives.

A systems biochemical understanding of the disease, the therapeutic agents' pharmacological properties (i.e., absorption, distribution, metabolism, excretion, and toxicity, or ADMET), and their functional impact on the human body both on-target and off-target would logically be necessary for the entire process, from target discovery to target validation to clinical testing and ultimately clinical adoption.

System biochemistry refers to the "global biochemical networks and molecular regulations". This is a challenging task for drug discovery, development, and its application using conventional methods, as is the case with all systems techniques. The effective and prosperous commercialization of promising therapeutic medicines is fundamentally hampered by the absence of systems biochemical methods and, consequently, functional understanding in the past. A systems biochemical understanding of the human body can now be envisioned for the first time due to the advancements in genomes, functional genomics, proteomics, and now metabolomics. Once created, this will hasten the knowledge of disease mechanisms and the creation of therapeutics at a rate never before seen. Comprehension of the biology of disease requires a thorough understanding of metabolism in human disorders. The metabolome is an essential component of molecular homeostasis regulation. Metabolomics, or the investigation of the metabolome, is currently being utilized for treating a wide range of disorders, mostly through metabolite profiling for biomarker discovery [2].

In recent years, the rapidly developing discipline of metabolomics has taken on a significant role due to its numerous applications in the area of drug discovery and development. Metabolomics has recently made significant strides, and it may now be used as a key tool in the process of finding and developing new drugs.

2. Metabolomics and its evolution

Dr. David Wishart's Human Metabolome Project has completed a year of study on the human metabolome, which contains 2500 metabolites, 1200 medicines, and 3500 dietary components. The $7.5 million research recruited 53 scientists and archived findings on the Human Metabolome Database. The study employs cutting-edge techniques such as NMR spectroscopy, mass spectrometry, multidimensional chromatography, and machine learning to profile metabolites without bias and characterize metabolite interactions using multivariate methodologies [3]. Professor Jeremy Nicholson first put up the idea of metabolomics in 1999. Using a similar principle to genomics and proteomics, metabolomics is a method to quantitatively analyze all metabolites produced by organisms to determine their link to pathological and physiological changes [4, 5].

The substrates and end products of metabolism, known as metabolites, fuel vital cellular processes such as energy production and storage, signal transduction, and apoptosis. Metabolites can come from bacteria, xenobiotics, food, and other foreign sources as well as to being produced naturally by the host organism [6]. Metabolomics is the study of the organism's internal store of non-proteinaceous small molecules. A thorough examination of the entire metabolome (the sum of all the low molecular weight compounds that are present in cells during a specific physiological condition. It alludes to the list of molecules found in a particular organism) under a specific set of circumstances is called metabolomics. Metabolomics is the only technique that can quantify interactions between the genome, proteome, and the biological "wild card" known as the outside environment. The emerging field of genomic science is metabolomics. The metabolomic society correlates with other post-genomic sciences; ideally, metabolomic data sets will be merged with its other omic sciences to provide comprehensive views

DOI: http://dx.doi.org/10.5772/intechopen.112969

into the molecular processes of system biology. However, unlike genomics or proteomics, which concentrate on characterizing huge macromolecules (DNA, RNA, and proteins), metabolomics concentrates on characterizing the small molecule, catabolic, and metabolic products resulting from the interactions of these large molecule [7].

3. Metabolomic study design

Metabolomics experiment involves Experimental design, sample collection and preparation, sample analysis, data processing, and interpretation (**Figure 1**).

3.1 Experimental design

A proper experimental design is crucial for accurate interpretation of data, including sufficient subjects, matching covariates, proper sample collection, and appropriate data analysis techniques [9].

3.1.1 Sample collection and preparation

Metabolic profiling analyses metabolites in both vivo and vitro samples. Metabolomics can analyze various biological materials, including biofluids, cells, tissue, and feces [10]. Standardized procedures for sample collection and storage improve

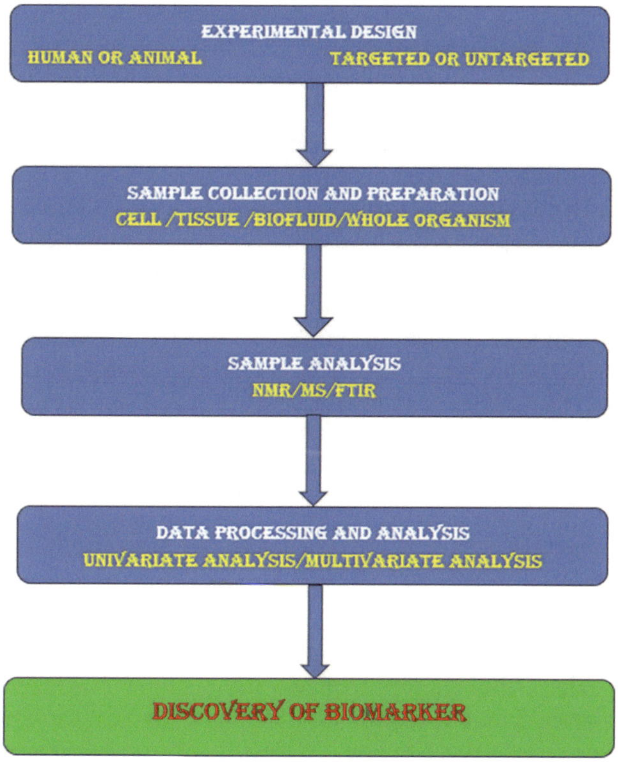

Figure 1.
Metabolomic workflow [8]. **Note:** *NMR (nuclear magnetic resonance), MS (mass spectroscopy), FTIR (Fourier transform infrared spectroscopy).*

quality and reproducibility. Factors like fed vs. fasting state, medications, blood collection time and processing time, addition of additives and potential sample hemolysis considerations can affect metabolites, leading to false-positive or false-negative results. Sample preparation depends on the analytical approaches to be utilized for analysis, such as NMR approaches requiring less preparation as a result it does not affect the sample much whereas mass spectrometry-based approaches requiring sample extraction by using different solvents. Metabolomics studies examine metabolites at specific time points, enabling more dynamic assessments of specific metabolic pathways. Recent development by introducing metabolite with isotope (13C) allows dynamic assessment of metabolic pathways, determining intracellular molecule sources, metabolite fate, flux, and cellular redox balance, providing details information which are not available in case of steady-state metabolomics experiments [10–14].

Sample pretreatment plays an important role. Pretreatment separation modalities include gas chromatography for gas phase separation of molecules useful in the analysis of traces of volatile compounds in samples, high performance liquid chromatography allows high pressure elution that leads to increase in the chromatographic separation of the samples makes it more versatile separation technique, capillary electrophoresis works on the principle of electrokinetic separation useful in the separation of small inorganic ions to larger proteins. These techniques offer advantages in characterizing specific aspects of a metabolome [15].

3.2 Detection methods

Targeted and untargeted metabolomic analyses are the two main categories that can be used, in theory. Targeted analysis would concentrate on a certain number of identified compounds. Untargeted metabolomics, also known as discovery metabolomics, tries to gather all the metabolomic data in a sample, while In the latter, features of relevance are identified after being filtered using various uni and multi-variate statistical techniques following data capture [16].

For the isolation and quantification of metabolome components, a wide range of targeted and untargeted approaches have already been documented in the literature. It was discovered, however, that no one analytical platform is able to collect complete metabolomics data in a single run (**Figure 2**) [17].

Metabolic profiling manly based upon the two specialized analytical techniques viz. NMR spectroscopy and MS. These techniques are efficient enough to identify and quantify wide range of molecules requiring small amount of sample. NMR spectroscopy based on the frequency pattern resulting from the interaction of nuclei of the molecule with the electromagnetic field. This pattern can give the information such as structure of the molecule, its motion, and chemical environment [18]. The identification and measurement of metabolites utilizing NMR techniques, such as proton NMR, 13C NMR, 19F NMR, and 31P NMR spectroscopy, have improved recently. The development of cryoprobes and microprobes, which have decreased the detection limit by a factor of around 3 to 5, is noteworthy. This approach is further enhanced by using two-dimensional total correlation spectroscopy (2D TOCSY) for the confirmation of assigned peaks. Other examples of two-dimensional NMR that have been used to enhance NMR-based data acquisition and metabolite structure analysis include Nuclear Overhauser effect spectroscopy (NOESY), heteronuclear single quantum coherence (HSQC), exchange spectroscopy (ES), and J spectroscopy (JS). These techniques provide better information than one-dimensional NMR, particularly for small-molecule metabolites. Furthermore, better outcome in the metabolome

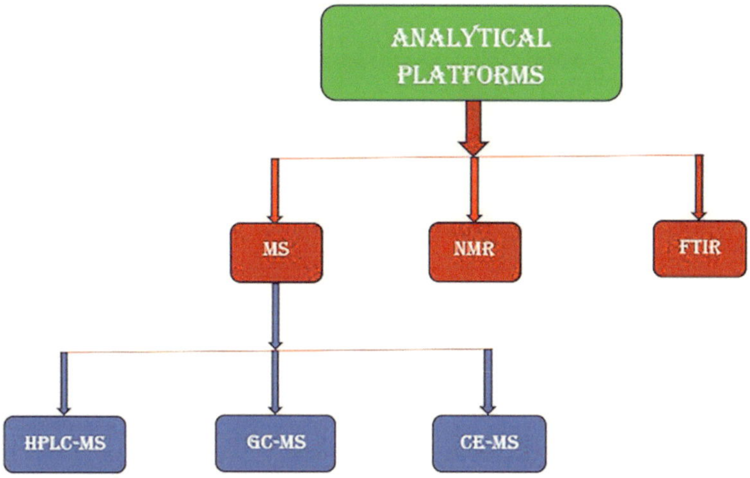

Figure 2.
Major analytical platforms for metabolomic studies in human and animal samples. **Note:** *HPLC (high performance liquid chromatography), GC (gas chromatography), CE (capillary electrophoresis).*

analysis can be achieved by the combination of 2D NMRs such as NOESY and HSQC and TOQCY and HSQC, by combining with MS with NMR or by 3DNMR [8]. NMR spectroscopy is rapid, non-destructive and gives reproducible results which makes its most reliable. Furthermore, samples that have undergone NMR analysis may undergo subsequent MS analysis. This technology's shortcomings are its lack of sensitivity and high user obtaining the necessary tools comes at a significant initial start-up cost and requires special training [19]. In contrast, the destructive analytical method known as mass spectrometry relies on the production of gas phase ions that are then distinguished by their charge/mass ratio. The number of ions for each mass/charge ratio is then calculated once the ions have reached the detector. In order to determine the molecular identities of the constituents, this is processed and compared against accessible mass spectral databases. MS is a very sensitive sample analysis technique that may be applied to both targeted and non-targeted analyses. However, the experimental setup and the instrument parameters have a significant impact on the detection's sensitivity and accuracy [18, 19].

The MS methodology is typically combined with chromatographic methods that have variable degrees of sensitivity, such as liquid chromatography (LC-MS), particularly high-performance liquid chromatography (HPLC- MS), and gas chromatography (GC-MS). Capillary electrophoresis and the MS method can also be combined for better outcome (CE-MS) [20].

A part from NMR and MS, FTIR is another tool which can be utilized successfully for metabolomic study (**Table 1**) [21].

3.3 Data analysis

This phase entails identifying metabolites and figuring out their relative abundance. The platform and method (targeted vs. untargeted) affects how metabolite identification occurs [23].

Standards are typically run in targeted studies and metabolite identification is less uncertain [24]. Whereas metabolite identification in the untargeted technique

Properties	Techniques			
	NMR	**HPLC-MS**	**CE-MS**	**GC-MS**
Sensitivity	–	++	+	+++
Reproducibility	High	Low	Low	Low
Resolution	Low	High	High	High
Quantity of sample requirement	Low	Medium	Medium	Extensive
Cost	Costly	Cost friendly	Cost friendly	Cost friendly
Range of metabolites	Polar and Non-Polar	RPLC: Non-Polar; HILIC: polar	Polar	Volatile polar and non-polar
Metabolite identification	Easy	Difficult (Database need to be improved)	Difficult (Database need to be improved)	Easy (Spectral libraries)

Note: *RPLC: Reverse Phase Liquid Chromatography; HILIC: Hydrophilic Interaction Liquid Chromatography [22].*

Table 1.
Comparison of commonly employed analytical techniques.

is uncertain comparatively, the spectra's are analyzed using either proprietary or publicly accessible software [25].

Additionally, the data should be checked for anomalies and samples or metabolites with a large number of missing values. Samples or metabolites that do not adhere to quality control standards should be eliminated at this stage. These actions result in the acquisition of a set of robustly measured metabolite [26, 27]. Rapid and precise statistical tools are required to handle the complexity and volume of the enormous amount of created data. For data analysis, several metabolomic features may be employed as the input. Spectral bin areas, metabolite concentrations, and spectral peak areas are some of these [28].

Numerous univariate and multivariate statistical methods can be used, focusing on data pre- and post-processing tasks such peak fitting, noise reduction, run order drift correction, and signal extraction/peak recognition. They are collectively referred to as chemometric approaches. The metabolomic characteristics are independently analyzed using univariate techniques [29]. Due to the fact that they use more widely accepted and understood statistical techniques, they are frequently simpler to interpret. However, the presence of interactions between various metabolic features is not taken into account in this approach. Confounding factors like gender, nutrition, or BMI are not taken into account. This raises the likelihood of receiving inaccurate results. Unlike univariate analysis, multivariate analysis takes into account all imputed metabolomic variables and attempts to uncover connections between them. These methods are divided into two categories: supervised methods and unsupervised methods. The most prevalent unsupervised method is principal component analysis, which is capable of detecting data patterns with biological variables. Supervised approaches find patterns within variables of interest while ignoring other sources of variation. Partial least squares regression analysis is the most commonly used supervised statistical procedure [30].

There are a number of software tools available for doing metabolite set enrichment analysis and visualizing the results. Metaboanalyst (www.metaboanalyst.ca)

is a website for metabolomics data analysis, which includes many tools for pathway enrichment analysis [31]. Metlin (https://metlin.scripps.edu), a massive database of metabolites with their MS-derived ions that serve for creative pathway analysis, is an online platform that allows extensive analyses and interpretation of omics data [9]. Metabox (free at http://kwanjeeraw.github.io/metabox/) (retrieved on January 10, 2020) under the GPL-3 license) [32] and MetaboAnalyst (http://www.metaboanalyst.ca/MetaboAnalyst [accessed: January 10, 2020]) [22]. Others such as SECIMTools, Meta XCMS, XCMS, XCMS2, MetAlign, MZmine for MS data processing, and MetDAT for statistical analysis and pathway visualization are among the tools available [8].

4. Metabolomics in the drug discovery and development

Drug research has become increasingly expensive, challenging, and risky over the previous two decades. The costs of research and development have risen, as has the cost of bringing a novel medicine through all stages of testing, which has a direct impact on the frequency with which a new drug is launched to the market. This is because pharmaceutical companies are unable to identify the therapeutic target or because of the multiple targets in case of complicated diseases such as cancer, heart disease, obesity, Alzheimer's disease etc. Another key issue is that the rate of converting a promising lead to a drug is decreasing; just one out of every thirty lead compounds reaches phase-I clinical trials, and only one out of every six drugs crosses clinical trials and enters the market. Still, there is a 5% chance that the drug may be withdrawn from the market due to adverse occurrences. Such failures can be costly for pharmaceutical corporations, affecting drug pricing directly. These failures can be addressed or reduced by strengthening drug target screening, tracking drug toxicity in the preclinical or developmental stage, and monitoring and reporting ADRs during the prescription or physician stage. Metabolomics, an emerging discipline of Omics science, can help to mitigate such failures and accelerate the drug discovery process [33–35]. In recent development ADME studies are commonly employed in drug discovery to optimize the balance of attributes required to turn leads into safe drugs. Metabolite characterization has recently emerged as a key driver in the drug discovery process, assisting in the optimisation of ADME characteristics and increasing drug success rates. For decades, it has been a valuable and important aspect of the drug development process. Over the last decade, there has been an increased effort to solve metabolic concerns using high throughput technologies for screening compounds, which has resulted in a strong need for more quick approaches for metabolite identification [7]. It has been discovered that metabolomics can provide drug researchers and regulators with an efficient and cost-effective method for discovering and developing viable medicinal products (**Figure 3**).

Metabolomics could aid in the following areas of drug discovery and development process:

4.1 Lead compound identification

Metabolomics, natural product chemistry and synthetic medicinal chemistry mainly focusses on the identification and characterization of small molecules as maximum of the FDA approved drugs are small molecules with a molecular weight (≤1500 Da) [37]. It is estimated that majority of these approved drugs are of pre-existing metabolites or preexisting natural product in nature (few examples such as

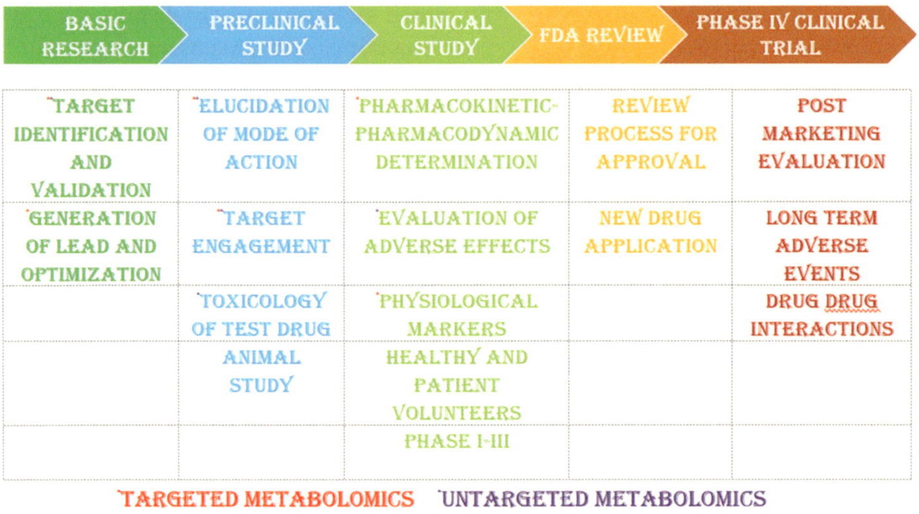

Figure 3.
Application of metabolomics in drug discovery and development [36].

corticosteroids and their derivatives to treat inflammation, ascorbic acid from citrus fruit to treat scurvy, quinine from cinchona tree to treat malaria, paclitaxel from yew bark to treat breast cancer etc.).It has been observed that small molecules are cofactors or substrates for at least one third of human proteins, hence identifying the unexplored ones from plant and human could become an excellent source for new drug candidates or drug scaffolds. Combination of experimental, computational and bibliographic surveys are underway to identify and characterize new or little-known metabolites that plays important roles in cell physiology, enzymatic activity, stress response and disease [38, 39]. Prior metabolite knowledge about known or hypothetical compounds is used in conjunction with NMR or MS data to identify novel compounds which are similar to currently available molecules. More than 20 million NMR and MS libraries of compounds are now available online can have impact on identification of new metabolite [40].

4.2 Lead prioritization and optimization

A number of leads will be generated as a result of any screening programme. One of the most important considerations in the drug development process is deciding which lead to prioritize. Compounds can be prioritized via metabolic profiling based on their capacity to generate the desired biochemical changes. Prioritization is now based on response strength and theoretical considerations of metabolism and toxicity. An inaccurate guess at this time could lead to the failure of the entire programme. A metabolomic analysis can help to distinguish the leads based on their primary and secondary reactions.

In order to progress from a lead to a therapeutic candidate, the lead is employed as a basis structure for the synthesis of hundreds of derivatives in a process known as "lead optimisation." In this step, chemists make several changes to the initial lead and test the impact of the alterations on activity. Each lead is assigned a metabolic profile, and the lead is optimized depending on the profile. This procedure is continued until the final lead candidate with the fewest secondary effects is chosen [41–44].

4.3 Target identification and validation

Identifying bioactive molecule targets is a major difficulty in chemical biological research. Metabolons, a proprietary technology platform, allows researchers to precisely gauge the multitude of metabolic alterations inherent in a specific disease and then map these changes to known pathways, helping them to better understand the disease.to establish a biochemical hypothesis for an ailment quickly. Based on this concept, illness-causing enzymes and proteins can be identified, and druggable disease targets can be located [7]. There are two basic methods for identifying chemical inhibitor targets: direct and indirect. The target proteins bound to the inhibitor are isolated and immediately identified by mass spectrometry in the direct technique. The indirect technique to identifying chemical inhibitor targets is searching for candidates by profiling biological data. If the drug was discovered to disrupt some cellular event for which the regulatory signaling pathway is known, targets can be identified by studying the compound's influence on each stage of the pathway. In some circumstances, omics research (for example, proteomics, transcriptomics, and metabolomics) can aid in the thorough analysis of a compound's effect on a potentially huge number of biological stages. Metabolomic profiling approaches gives the information about the biochemical fingerprint for a specific target. The target can be biochemically validated by identifying any unanticipated adverse effects and by comparing the target to the disease itself. It is also feasible to discover unanticipated secondary effects inherent in a target, so as to discard a target that may pose prohibitive risk [45, 46].

4.4 Biomarker identification

Being able to quantitatively detect, measure, or monitor the disease for which the medicine is being created is crucial to drug development. A medicine to treat a disease cannot be produced until the disease is measured. Many of today's disease assays and diagnostic tests utilize small molecules (i.e., Metabolite) biomarkers as indicators of disease or condition (absence/presence/severity). Metabolomics is primarily concerned with the detection and quantification of small molecule biomarkers (i.e., biomarkers for disease and therapeutic efficacy). Metabolomics has already been used to identify small molecule biomarkers or multi-metabolite signatures for a wide range of diseases such as hypertension, heart failure, Parkinson's disease, prostate cancer, breast cancer, ovarian cancer, schizophrenia, Alzheimer's disease, and coronary heart disease, etc. [47–56]. The most successful application of metabolomics is to discover inborn errors of metabolism (IEMs), with NMR-based metabolomics capable of identifying and monitoring more than 85 different IEMs and MS-based metabolomics capable of detecting and monitoring 130 different IEMs. (For example, phenylketonuria can be diagnosed by low tyrosine levels, Tay Sachs disease by high GM2 ganglioside levels, and cystinuria by high lysine and cystine levels.) [36, 57].

4.5 Mode of action

The justification of MoA using metabolomics usually demands prior information on the impacted metabolic pathways. In other words, drug-induced metabolic changes are statistically analyzed using route maps, and the most significantly affected nodes (proteins) are then selected for additional investigation/validation. This type of analysis can be performed by combining untargeted metabolomics with in silico or chemoinformatic techniques [58]. It can be utilized to predict not just the mode of action of the drug, but also the harmful mechanism of action [7].

4.6 Measuring drug metabolism

ADME testing is one of the most important aspects of drug development process. The process is very time consuming, expensive and error-prone [59]. The emergence high throughput metabolomic methods has opened up a new avenue for experimentally monitoring ADME and identifying metabolites and metabolic pathways associated with drug metabolism [60]. Methods for identifying drugs or drug metabolites rely more directly on experimental data analysis and spectral comparisons of dosed and un-dosed bio samples. These include mass defect filtering techniques [61] and multivariate data analysis of LC-MS chromatograms for MS and STOCSY for NMR spectroscopy, which can be used in conjunction with high resolution MS instruments such as FTICR (Fourier Transform Ion Cyclotron Resonance) or OrbitrapTM [60] spectrometers to generate exact molecular formulas. Compound identification is clearly only a subset of what is usually necessary for full ADME experiments. It is crucial to measure the amount, distribution, and location of a substance once it has been identified. It is also crucial to compare these results to those of other metabolites over time and space, and to conduct these measurements using additional biological or technical replicas. Fortunately, the high-throughput characteristic of most metabolomics technologies enables these multicomponent, multi-sample analyses to be carried out with great repeatability and at a reasonable cost [61].

4.7 Preclinical study

Metabolomics approaches can be applied rapidly and noninvasively in a number of toxicological assays such as Identification of target organ or region of toxicity, identification of biochemical mechanism of toxicity, identification and quantification of biomarkers profile which measure toxic effects, measurement of time course of toxic effects [62]. This can be employed as a safety screening mechanism by many pharmaceutical companies as an alternative to expensive and time-consuming toxicological and histopathological screening. Furthermore, it can be utilized to find toxicity biomarkers as a result of the identification of various biomarkers utilizing this platform [63].

4.8 Clinical study

Clinical trial monitoring and screening is very important in the drug discovery and development process. Clinical trial monitoring not only involves the effect of drug but also involves the influence of diet, drug use/abuse and behavioral factors on the outcome. Metabolomics can be can be useful in-patient monitoring by detecting the presence of over-the-counter drugs, herbal supplements, drugs of abuse and food by products in clinical trials settings to assure patients compliance [64–67]. This method be useful in the patient screening and drug patient matching. This approach can be utilized to examine drug metabolism characteristics in individual patients. There is significant diversity in patient responses to specific classes of medicines (such as antidepressants), which is largely owing to differences in drug metabolism profiles [68]. Certainly, detecting susceptible/refractory patients prior to recruitment (in clinical trials) or prescription (in clinical practice) would improve outcomes. The use of metabolomic-based phenotyping in clinical trials or drug dosage in clinical practise has the potential to be a quick and low-cost screening method for patient selection or drug dosing. These metabolomic assays would almost certainly be far less expensive in terms of both time and money than traditional approaches. Metabolomics is extremely effective in monitoring drug doses of relatively toxic pharmaceuticals (anticancer drugs such as methotrexate, 6-mercaptopurine, 5-flurouracil, etc., blood thinning agents such as warfarin, immunosuppressants such as mycophenolic acid and ciclosporin). Furthermore, it plays a critical role in detecting and monitoring ADRs, which are a huge burden for the pharmaceutical business and healthcare system (due to patient death and hospitalization). Endogenous metabolite levels in the blood and urine can be used to detect many undesirable medication effects [61].

5. Challenges for metabolomics

Data analysis is one of the most difficult aspects of metabolomics research. Metabolomics provides enormous volumes of data, often with complicated structures and patterns that necessitate the use of advanced computer techniques to analyze.

A second difficulty is sample deterioration and standardization. Metabolomics is a young discipline with few widely agreed standards for sample collection, processing, and analysis. Importantly, after a sample is extracted, its metabolic signature may differ from what it was in the biological system. This emphasizes the importance of sample preparation and makes comparing results between research and replicating trials challenging.

Another issue is the existing metabolomics techniques' lack of sensitivity and specificity. Despite substantial technological breakthroughs, contemporary metabolomics techniques are still incapable of detecting all metabolites in a given sample. This can result in false negatives or incorrect results [69].

6. Conclusion

Metabolomic principles have the potential to revolutionize the drug discovery and development process. Metabolomics focuses on the small molecules that are essential for life to exist and act as the molecular foundation for cells by supplying fuel for cellular processes. Small molecules also help to preserve cellular integrity, fights environmental stress, and acts as a cellular messenger for a variety of cellular activities. Drug discovery is a time-consuming, high-risk, and tremendously expensive procedure. Metabolic profiling is a sensitive indicator of phenotypic alterations as well as pharmacological on and off target of drug candidates. High-resolution metabolic profiling is possible using minimal sample preparation, and as part of various drug testing processes. Metabolomics can also offer drug selection markers that can be employed *in vivo* which are phenotypic specific.

Metabolomics allows scientists to investigate the known roles of small molecule metabolites in greater detail and with better precision than ever before. The increasing breadth of available coverage, increased sensitivity, greatly improved analytical software, and trends towards more accurate quantification enable certain types of novel metabolomics experiments that were only a dream a few years ago. Continuing development in the field metabolomics along the growing investment by the pharmaceutical industry players and FDA will foster a rapid and more cost-effective drug discovery and development process.

Acknowledgements

I would like to acknowledge the lab mates of Antimalarial Drug Discovery lab, Department of Pharmaceutical Sciences, Dibrugarh University, Assam, India.

Conflict of interest

The authors declare no conflict of interest.

Author details

Dipankar Nath* and Dipak Chetia
Department of Pharmaceutical Sciences, Dibrugarh University, Dibrugarh, India

*Address all correspondence to: pharmchem1209@gmail.com

References

[1] Ratti E, Trist D. Continuing evolution of the drug discovery process in the pharmaceutical industry. Pure and Applied Chemistry. 2001;**73**(1):67-75. DOI: 10.1351/pac200173010067

[2] Fan TW, Lorkiewicz PK, Sellers K, Moseley HN, Higashi RM, Lane AN. Stable isotope-resolved metabolomics and applications for drug development. Pharmacology & Therapeutics. 2012;**133**(3):366-391. DOI: 10.1016/j.pharmthera.2011.12.007

[3] Kasture VS, Musmade DS, Vakte MB, Sonawane SB, Patil PP. Metabolomics: Current technologies and future trends. International Journal of Research and Development in Pharmacy & Life Sciences (IJRDPL). 2012;**2**:206-217

[4] Nicholson JK, Lindon JC, Holmes E. 'Metabonomics': Understanding the metabolic responses of living systems to pathophysiological stimuli via multivariate statistical analysis of biological NMR spectroscopic data. Xenobiotica. 1999;**29**(11):1181-1189. DOI: 10.1080/004982599238047

[5] Andrew Clayton T, Lindon JC, Cloarec O, Antti H, Charuel C, Hanton G, et al. Pharmaco-metabonomic phenotyping and personalized drug treatment. Nature. 2006;**440**(7087):1073-1077. DOI: 10.1038/nature04648

[6] Johnson CH, Ivanisevic J, Siuzdak G. Metabolomics: Beyond biomarkers and towards mechanisms. Nature Reviews Molecular Cell Biology. 2016;**17**(7):451-459. DOI: 10.1038/nrm.2016.25

[7] Martis A, Ahire C, Ruchi S. Metabolomics in drug discovery: A review. International Journal of Pharmacy and Pharmaceutical Science Research. 2011;**1**:67-74

[8] Aderemi AV, Ayeleso AO, Oyedapo OO, Mukwevho E. Metabolomics: A scoping review of its role as a tool for disease biomarker discovery in selected non-communicable diseases. Metabolites. 2021;**11**(7):418. DOI: 10.3390/metabo11070418

[9] Liu Z, Waters J, Rui B. Metabolomics as a promising tool for improving understanding of multiple sclerosis: A review of recent advances. Biomedical Journal. 2022;**45**(4):594-606. DOI: 10.1016/j.bj.2022.01.004

[10] Chetwynd AJ, Dunn WB, Rodriguez-Blanco G. Collection and preparation of clinical samples for metabolomics. Advances in Experimental Medicine and Biology. 2017;**965**:19-44. DOI: 10.1007/978-3-319-47656-8_2

[11] Yin P, Peter A, Franken H, Zhao X, Neukamm SS, Rosenbaum L, et al. Preanalytical aspects and sample quality assessment in metabolomics studies of human blood. Clinical Chemistry. 2013;**59**(5):833-845. DOI: 10.1373/clinchem.2012.199257

[12] Pinto J, Domingues MR, Galhano E, Pita C, do Céu Almeida M, Carreira IM, Gil AM. Human plasma stability during handling and storage: Impact on NMR metabolomics. The Analyst. 2014;**139**(5):1168-1177. DOI: 10.1039/c3an02188b

[13] Zhang Z, Shen T, Rui B, Zhou W, Zhou X, Shang C, et al. CeCaFDB: A curated database for the documentation, visualization and comparative analysis of central carbon metabolic flux distributions explored by 13C-fluxomics. Nucleic Acids

Research. 2015;**43**(D1):D549-D557. DOI: 10.1093/nar/gku1137

[14] Ibrahim SM, Gold R. Genomics, proteomics, metabolomics: What is in a word for multiple sclerosis? Current Opinion in Neurology. 2005;**18**(3):231-235. DOI: 10.1097/01.wco.0000169738.06664.3b

[15] Ashrafian H, Sounderajah V, Glen R, Ebbels T, Blaise BJ, Kalra D, et al. Metabolomics: The stethoscope for the twenty-first century. Medical Principles and Practice. 2021;**30**(4):301-310. DOI: 10.1159/000513545

[16] Steuer AE, Brockbals L, Kraemer T. Metabolomic strategies in biomarker research–new approach for indirect identification of drug consumption and sample manipulation in clinical and forensic toxicology? Frontiers in Chemistry. 2019;7:319. DOI: 10.3389/fchem.2019.00319

[17] Dinis-Oliveira RJ. Metabolomics of drugs of abuse: A more realistic view of the toxicological complexity. Bioanalysis. 2014;**6**(23):3155-3159. DOI: 10.4155/bio.14.260

[18] Markley JL, Brüschweiler R, Edison AS, Eghbalnia HR, Powers R, Raftery D, et al. The future of NMR-based metabolomics. Current Opinion in Biotechnology. 2017;**43**:34-40. DOI: 10.1016/j.copbio.2016.08.001

[19] Gowda GA, Djukovic D. Overview of mass spectrometry-based metabolomics: opportunities and challenges. Methods in Molecular Biology. 2014;**1198**:3-12. DOI: 10.1007/978-1-4939-1258-2_1

[20] Mosana M, Ayeleso A, Nyakudya T, Erlwanger K, Mukwevho E. Potential protective effects of neonatal supplementation with oleanolic acid on peroxisome proliferator-activated receptor gamma (PPARγ)-ligand dependent regulation of glucose homeostasis in high fructose-fed rats. Natural Product Communications. 2020;**15**(3):1934578X20913747. DOI: 10.1177/1934578X20913747

[21] Armitage EG, Southam AD. Monitoring cancer prognosis, diagnosis and treatment efficacy using metabolomics and lipidomics. Metabolomics. 2016;**12**:1-5. DOI: 10.1007/s11306-016-1093-7

[22] Munjal Y, Tonk RK, Sharma R. Analytical techniques used in metabolomics: A review. Systematic Reviews in Pharmacy. 2022;**13**(5):515-521. DOI: 10.31858/0975-8453

[23] Cajka T, Fiehn O. Toward merging untargeted and targeted methods in mass spectrometry-based metabolomics and lipidomics. Analytical Chemistry. 2016;**88**(1):524-545. DOI: 10.1021/acs.analchem.5b04491

[24] Griffiths WJ, Koal T, Wang Y, Kohl M, Enot DP, Deigner HP. Targeted metabolomics for biomarker discovery. Angewandte Chemie International Edition. 2010;**49**(32):5426-5445. DOI: 10.1002/anie.200905579

[25] Schrimpe-Rutledge AC, Codreanu SG, Sherrod SD, McLean JA. Untargeted metabolomics strategies—Challenges and emerging directions. Journal of the American Society for Mass Spectrometry. 2016;**27**(12):1897-1905. DOI: 10.1007/s13361-016-1469-y

[26] Stoessel D, Stellmann JP, Willing A, Behrens B, Rosenkranz SC, Hodecker SC, et al. Metabolomic profiles for primary progressive multiple sclerosis stratification and disease course monitoring. Frontiers in Human Neuroscience. 2018;**12**:226. DOI: 10.3389/fnhum.2018.00226

[27] Nourbakhsh B, Bhargava P, Tremlett H, Hart J, Graves J, Waubant E. Altered tryptophan metabolism is associated with pediatric multiple sclerosis risk and course. Annals of Clinical and Translational Neurology. 2018;**5**(10):1211-1221. DOI: 10.1002/acn3.637

[28] Alonso A, Marsal S, Julià A. Analytical methods in untargeted metabolomics: State of the art in 2015. Frontiers in Bioengineering and Biotechnology. 2015;**3**:23. DOI: 10.3389/fbioe.2015.00023

[29] Putri SP, Yamamoto S, Tsugawa H, Fukusaki E. Current metabolomics: Technological advances. Journal of Bioscience and Bioengineering. 2013;**116**(1):9-16. DOI: 10.1016/j.jbiosc.2013.01.004

[30] Worley B, Powers R. Multivariate analysis in metabolomics. Current Metabolomics. 2013;**1**(1):92-107. DOI: 10.2174/2213235X11301010092

[31] Zhu XR, Yang FY, Lu J, Zhang HR, Sun R, Zhou JB, et al. Plasma metabolomic profiling of proliferative diabetic retinopathy. Nutrition & Metabolism. 2019;**16**(1):1-1. DOI: 10.1186/s12986-019-0358-3

[32] Yilmaz A, Geddes T, Han B, Bahado-Singh RO, Wilson GD, Imam K, et al. Diagnostic biomarkers of Alzheimer's disease as identified in saliva using 1H NMR-based metabolomics. Journal of Alzheimer's Disease. 2017;**58**(2):355-359. DOI: 10.3233/JAD-161226

[33] DiMasi JA, Hansen RW, Grabowski HG. The price of innovation: New estimates of drug development costs. Journal of Health Economics. 2003;**22**(2):151-185. DOI: 10.1016/S0167-6296(02)00126-1

[34] Frantz S. Pipeline problems are increasing the urge to merge. Nature Reviews Drug Discovery. 2006;**5**(12):977-979. DOI: 10.1038/nrd2206

[35] Wishart DS. Applications of metabolomics in drug discovery and development. Drugs in R&D. 2008;**9**:307-322. DOI: 10.2165/00126839-200809050-00002

[36] Alarcon-Barrera JC, Kostidis S, Ondo-Mendez A, Giera M. Recent advances in metabolomics analysis for early drug development. Drug Discovery Today. 2022;**27**(6):1763-1773. DOI: 10.1016/j.drudis.2022.02.018

[37] Wishart DS, Knox C, Guo AC, Shrivastava S, Hassanali M, Stothard P, et al. Drugbank: A comprehensive resource for in silico drug discovery and exploration. Nucleic Acids Research. 2006;**34**(suppl 1):D668-D672. DOI: 10.1093/nar/gkj067

[38] Newman DJ, Cragg GM. Natural products as sources of new drugs over the last 25 years. Journal of Natural Products. 2007;**70**(3):461-477. DOI: 10.1021/np068054v

[39] Wishart DS, Knox C, Guo AC, Eisner R, Young N, Gautam B, et al. HMDB: A knowledgebase for the human metabolome. Nucleic Acids Research. 2009;**37**(suppl_1):D603-D610. DOI: 10.1093/nar/gkn810

[40] Cloarec O, Dumas ME, Craig A, Barton RH, Trygg J, Hudson J, et al. Statistical total correlation spectroscopy: An exploratory approach for latent biomarker identification from metabolic 1H NMR data sets. Analytical Chemistry. 2005;**77**(5):1282-1289. DOI: 10.1021/ac048630x

[41] Nicholson JK, Connelly J, Lindon JC, Holmes E. Metabonomics:

A platform for studying drug toxicity and gene function. Nature Reviews Drug Discovery. 2002;**1**(2):153-161. DOI: 10.1038/nrd728

[42] Watkins SM, German JB. Metabolomics and biochemical profiling in drug discovery and development. Current Opinion in Molecular Therapeutics. 2002;**4**(3):224-228

[43] Wang M, Lamers RJ, Korthout HA, van Nesselrooij JH, Witkamp RF, van der Heijden R, et al. Metabolomics in the context of systems biology: Bridging traditional Chinese medicine and molecular pharmacology. Phytotherapy Research. 2005;**19**(3):173-182. DOI: 10.1002/ptr.1624

[44] Xu EY, Schaefer WH, Xu Q. Metabolomics in pharmaceutical research and development: Metabolites, mechanisms and pathways. Current Opinion in Drug Discovery & Development. 2009;**12**(1):40-52

[45] Braaksma M, Bijlsma S, Coulier L, Punt PJ, van der Werf MJ. Metabolomics as a tool for target identification in strain improvement: The influence of phenotype definition. Microbiology. 2011;**157**(1):147-159. DOI: 10.1099/mic.0.041244-0

[46] Kitagawa M, Ikeda S, Tashiro E, Soga T, Imoto M. Metabolomic identification of the target of the filopodia protrusion inhibitor glucopiericidin a. Chemistry & Biology. 2010;**17**(9):989-998. DOI: 10.1016/j.chembiol.2010.06.017

[47] Tietz NW. Clinical Guide to Laboratory Tests. Philadelphia, PA, USA: W.B. Saunders, Co.; 1995. pp. 1096-1096

[48] Brindle JT, Nicholson JK, Schofield PM, Grainger DJ, Holmes E. Application of chemometrics to 1H NMR spectroscopic data to investigate a relationship between human serum metabolic profiles and hypertension. Analyst. Jan 2003;**128**(1):32-36. DOI: 10.1039/b209155k

[49] Dunn WB, Broadhurst DI, Deepak SM, Buch MH, McDowell G, Spasic I, et al. Serum metabolomics reveals many novel metabolic markers of heart failure, including pseudouridine and 2-oxoglutarate. Metabolomics. 2007;**3**:413-426. DOI: 10.1007/s11306-007-0063-5

[50] Bogdanov M, Matson WR, Wang L, Matson T, Saunders-Pullman R, Bressman SS, et al. Metabolomic profiling to develop blood biomarkers for Parkinson's disease. Brain. 2008;**131**(2):389-396. DOI: 10.1093/brain/awm304

[51] Serkova NJ, Gamito EJ, Jones RH, O'Donnell C, Brown JL, Green S, et al. The metabolites citrate, myo-inositol, and spermine are potential age-independent markers of prostate cancer in human expressed prostatic secretions. The Prostate. 2008;**68**(6):620-628. DOI: 10.1002/pros.20727

[52] Fan X, Bai J, Shen P. Diagnosis of breast cancer using HPLC metabonomics fingerprints coupled with computational methods. In: Conference Proceedings - IEEE Engineering in Medicine and Biology Society. Vol. 2005. 2005. pp. 6081-6084. DOI: 10.1109/IEMBS.2005.1615880

[53] Odunsi K, Wollman RM, Ambrosone CB, Hutson A, McCann SE, Tammela J, et al. Detection of epithelial ovarian cancer using 1H-NMR-based metabonomics. International Journal of Cancer. 2005;**113**(5):782-788. DOI: 10.1002/ijc.20651

[54] Kaddurah-Daouk R. Metabolic profiling of patients with schizophrenia. PLoS Medicine. 2006;**3**(8):e363. DOI: 10.1371/journal.pmed.0030363

[55] Han X, Holtzman M, McKeel DW Jr, Kelley J, Morris JC. Substantial sulfatide deficiency and ceramide elevation in very early Alzheimer's disease: Potential role in disease pathogenesis. Journal of Neurochemistry. 2002;**82**(4):809-818. DOI: 10.1046/j.1471-4159.2002.00997.x

[56] Brindle JT, Antti H, Holmes E, Tranter G, Nicholson JK, Bethell HW, et al. Rapid and noninvasive diagnosis of the presence and severity of coronary heart disease using 1H-NMR-based metabonomics. Nature Medicine. 2002;**8**(12):1439-1445. DOI: 10.1038/nm1202-802

[57] Moolenaar SH, Engelke UF, Wevers RA. Proton nuclear magnetic resonance spectroscopy of body fluids in the field of inborn errors of metabolism. Annals of Clinical Biochemistry. 2003;**40**(1):16-24. DOI: 10.1258/000456303321016132

[58] Kuhara T. Noninvasive human metabolome analysis for differential diagnosis of inborn errors of metabolism. Journal of Chromatography B. 2007;**855**(1):42-50. DOI: 10.1016/j.jchromb.2007.03.031

[59] Wishart DS. Improving early drug discovery through ADME modelling: An overview. Drugs in R&D. 2007;**8**:349-362. DOI: 10.2165/00126839-200708060-00003

[60] Chen C, Gonzalez FJ, Idle JR. LC-MS-based metabolomics in drug metabolism. Drug Metabolism Reviews. 2007;**39**(2-3):581-597. DOI: 10.1080/03602530701497804

[61] Wishart DS. Applications of metabolomics in drug discovery and development. Drugs in R&D. 2008;**9**(5):307-322. DOI: 10.2165/00126839-200809050-00002

[62] Lindon JC, Holmes E, Nicholson JK. Metabonomics in pharmaceutical R&D. The FEBS Journal. 2007;**274**(5):1140-1151. DOI: 10.1111/j.1742-4658.2007.05673.x

[63] Robertson DG, Reily MD, Baker JD. Metabonomics in pharmaceutical discovery and development. Journal of Proteome Research. 2007;**6**(2):526-539. DOI: 10.1021/pr060535c

[64] Holmes E, Loo RL, Cloarec O, Coen M, Tang H, Maibaum E, et al. Detection of urinary drug metabolite (xenometabolome) signatures in molecular epidemiology studies via statistical total correlation (NMR) spectroscopy. Analytical Chemistry. 2007;**79**(7):2629-2640. DOI: 10.1021/ac062305n

[65] Giri S, Idle JR, Chen C, Zabriskie TM, Krausz KW, Gonzalez FJ. A metabolomic approach to the metabolism of the areca nut alkaloids arecoline and arecaidine in the mouse. Chemical Research in Toxicology. 2006;**19**(6):818-827. DOI: 10.1021/tx0600402

[66] Mennen LI, Sapinho D, Ito H, Bertrais S, Galan P, Hercberg S, et al. Urinary flavonoids and phenolic acids as biomarkers of intake for polyphenol-rich foods. British Journal of Nutrition. 2006;**96**(1):191-198. DOI: 10.1079/bjn20061808

[67] Keun HC, Athersuch TJ. Application of metabonomics in drug development. Pharmacogenomics. 2007;**8**(7):731-741. DOI: 10.2217/14622416.8.7.731

[68] Thuerauf N, Lunkenheimer J. The impact of the CYP2D6-polymorphism on dose recommendations for current antidepressants. European Archives of Psychiatry and Clinical Neuroscience. 2006;**256**:287-293. DOI: 10.1007/s00406-006-0663-5

[69] Overcoming challenges and capitalizing on opportunities in metabolomics [Internet]. 2023. Available from: https://gigantest.com/article/overcoming-challenges-opportunities-metabolomics/

Chapter 5

The Role of Bioinformatics in Drug Discovery: A Comprehensive Overview

Dogfounianalo Somda, Stephen Wilson Kpordze, Mercy Jerpkorir, Mishell Chantelle Mahora, Jecinta Wanjiru Ndungu, Sally Wambui Kamau, Vera Arthur and Amel Elbasyouni

Abstract

Bioinformatics plays a crucial role in various aspects of drug discovery, drug metabolism, and pharmacology. In drug discovery, bioinformatics enables the efficient analysis and interpretation of large-scale biological data, facilitating target identification, lead compound optimization, and prediction of drug-target interactions. It aids in the identification and characterization of potential drug targets through genomic and proteomic analyses. Additionally, bioinformatics assists in the prediction of drug metabolism and pharmacokinetic properties, offering insights into the safety and efficacy of potential drug candidates. Furthermore, it contributes to pharmacology by enabling the analysis of drug-drug interactions, adverse drug reactions, and personalized medicine approaches. The integration of computational tools and algorithms with biological and chemical data has accelerated the drug discovery process, improved success rates, and reduced costs. Bioinformatics has become an indispensable tool in the development of novel therapeutics and the optimization of drug efficacy and safety. This book chapter elucidates the profound impact of bioinformatics in drug metabolism and pharmacology, emphasizing the transformative potential it holds for the future of pharmaceutical research, ultimately improving patient outcomes and bringing innovative therapies.

Keywords: bioinformatics, technology, drug metabolism, pharmacology, innovative, drug discovery

1. Introduction

The process of drug development is a complex and resource-intensive undertaking that is crucial to the pharmaceutical industry's objective of enhancing healthcare outcomes on a global scale. The endeavor encompasses a diverse range of experiences that last over an extended period, encompassing multiple phases, and necessitating significant financial resources [1]. Drug development is primarily motivated by the objective of developing therapies that are safer, more effective, and characterized by innovation, with the aim of addressing medical requirements that have not yet been satisfied [2].

The initial step is the identification of a specific chemical or pathway that is associated with a particular disease [3]. The commencement of this preliminary stage frequently arises from comprehensive biological investigation and a profound comprehension of the fundamental causes of the disease [3–6]. After the identification of a target, drug candidates are formulated, manufactured, and subjected to comprehensive laboratory testing. The initial preclinical phases involve evaluating the potential effectiveness and safety of the proposed drugs [7]. After successful selection, candidates progress to the clinical phase, which encompasses a series of human trials specifically designed to assess the safety, dose, and efficacy of the intervention. This phase is comprised of three distinct segments. Phase I trials typically encompass a limited number of individuals who are in good health, Phase II trials thereafter encompass a larger cohort of patients diagnosed with the specific ailment under investigation, and Phase III trials comprise an even more extensive and diverse patient population. Clinical trials are frequently characterized by their lengthy duration, substantial financial investment, and stringent regulatory oversight, all of which are implemented to safeguard the safety and effectiveness of the prospective pharmaceutical compound [8]. The process of regulatory submission is characterized by its stringent nature, necessitating the provision of comprehensive data pertaining to safety, efficacy, and manufacturing quality [9–11]. In conjunction with clinical trials, pharmaceutical corporations allocate significant resources toward research and development (R&D), which involves the employment of extensive teams comprising scientists, physicians, and support workers. In addition, researchers are required to effectively manage a multifaceted network of intellectual property concerns, wherein they engage in the process of patenting their findings as a means to safeguard their investments and establish market exclusivity.

The process from the identification of an objective through the attainment of regulatory approval is replete with many hurdles, encompassing the potential for failure at any given point. The majority of medication candidates fail to successfully complete the entire process, primarily owing to safety concerns, lack of efficacy, or other factors. The attrition rate, when coupled with the substantial expenses associated with clinical development, renders drug development a high-stakes and resource-intensive undertaking. Hence, the process of drug development is complex, time-consuming, and expensive, necessitating the integration of scientific knowledge, financial capital, regulatory supervision, and a steadfast dedication to enhancing worldwide healthcare. Despite the intricate nature and difficulties associated with it, the pharmaceutical sector continues to persist in its endeavor to develop innovative treatments that have the potential to revolutionize the quality of life and mitigate the impact of illnesses on the broader community.

With the rapid progress in technology, it is noteworthy that bioinformatics has emerged as an essential instrument in contemporary biological research. This field empowers scientists to get significant insights from extensive and intricate information. Bioinformatics is an interdisciplinary domain situated at the convergence of biology, computer science, and data analysis. The field encompasses the utilization of computational methodologies and statistical approaches to effectively handle, scrutinize, and elucidate biological information [12, 13]. The aforementioned discipline holds significant importance in multiple domains of biology, encompassing genomics, proteomics, evolutionary biology, and drug development. This book chapter provides a comprehensive examination of the pivotal role that bioinformatics plays in the realms of drug metabolism and pharmacology.

2. Bioinformatics in drug metabolism

The process of drug metabolism holds significant importance in the field of pharmaceutical research and development, as it governs the ultimate disposition of pharmaceuticals within the human body. The field of bioinformatics assumes a pivotal function in comprehending and enhancing the mechanisms of drug metabolism. Bioinformatics plays a pivotal role in advancing drug metabolism research through several significant avenues (**Figure 1**) [12, 13].

The prediction of metabolic pathways involves the utilization of bioinformatics techniques and databases to anticipate the potential metabolic transformations that a medication may undergo within the physiological context of the human body [14–18]. The aforementioned is crucial in evaluating the safety and effectiveness

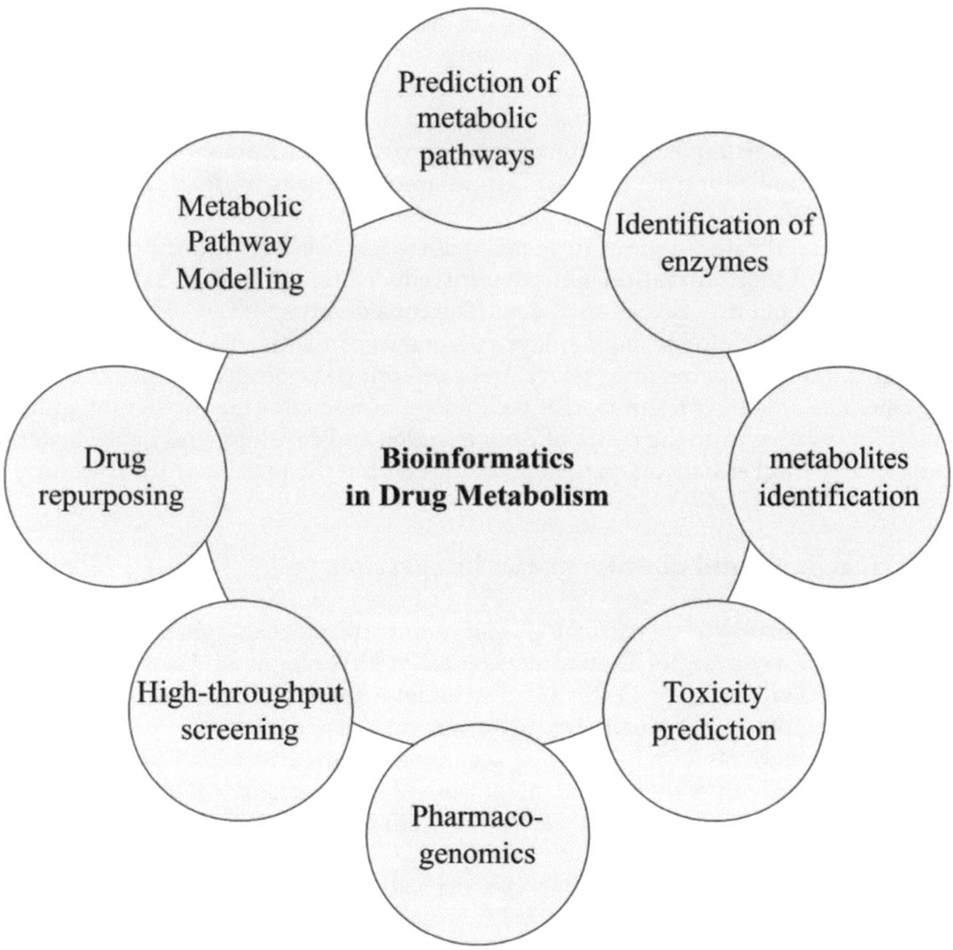

Figure 1.
Application of bioinformatics in drug metabolism.

of a pharmaceutical compound under consideration [12, 19–24]. The utilization of bioinformatics facilitates the identification of distinct enzymes that play a role in the process of drug metabolism. The identification of the specific enzymes involved in the metabolism of a drug is of utmost importance in the anticipation of drug-drug interactions and the potential manifestation of adverse effects. The utilization of bioinformatics tools facilitates the process of identifying and characterizing drug metabolites. Metabolites possess distinct pharmacological characteristics in comparison to the original drug, and their identification is crucial for assessing the comprehensive effects of a medication. The utilization of bioinformatics models enables the prediction of probable harmful metabolites or drug metabolism products, hence facilitating the evaluation of the safety profile of drug candidates by researchers.

The field of pharmacogenomics investigates genetic differences in drug-metabolizing enzymes across diverse populations. The aforementioned data is used to individualize pharmaceutical interventions, hence guaranteeing that individuals are administered the most efficacious and secure medications in accordance with their genetic characteristics [25].

Bioinformatics tools play a crucial role in the analysis of high-throughput screening data for drug discovery. These tools assist in the identification of prospective medication candidates and the prioritization of compounds for subsequent testing, utilizing their metabolic profiles. Drug repurposing, a process facilitated by bioinformatics, involves the analysis of metabolic pathways and the identification of potential off-target effects of existing medications, leading to the discovery of novel therapeutic applications. The implementation of this approach has the potential to expedite the process of medication development while simultaneously mitigating financial expenditures [26–28].

In summary, the discipline of drug metabolism has been significantly transformed by the advent of bioinformatics, which has introduced robust tools and procedures for the analysis and interpretation of data. The consideration of individual genetic differences in medication response plays a pivotal role in optimizing drug development processes, enhancing drug safety, and promoting the progress of personalized medicine. The ongoing progression of technology necessitates the further integration of bioinformatics within the realm of drug research and development, hence fostering innovation and enhancing patient outcomes within the pharmaceutical sector.

3. Pharmacology and bioinformatics integration

The amalgamation of pharmacology and bioinformatics exemplifies a potent synergy between conventional pharmacological methodologies and state-of-the-art computational tools [23, 25, 29–32]. The integration of bioinformatics in drug development pipeline has greatly improved our capacity to identify, create, and refine pharmaceuticals with heightened accuracy and effectiveness. This part of the chapter provides an overview of the integration of pharmacology and bioinformatics, highlighting its transformative impact on the domain of drug discovery and development (**Figure 2**).

First, bioinformatics tools facilitate the methodical examination of biological data encompassing genomes, proteomics, and transcriptomics, with the aim of identifying and validating new therapeutic targets [33–36]. Through the examination of extensive datasets, researchers have the ability to identify particular genes, proteins, or pathways that assume critical functions in the development and progression of diseases.

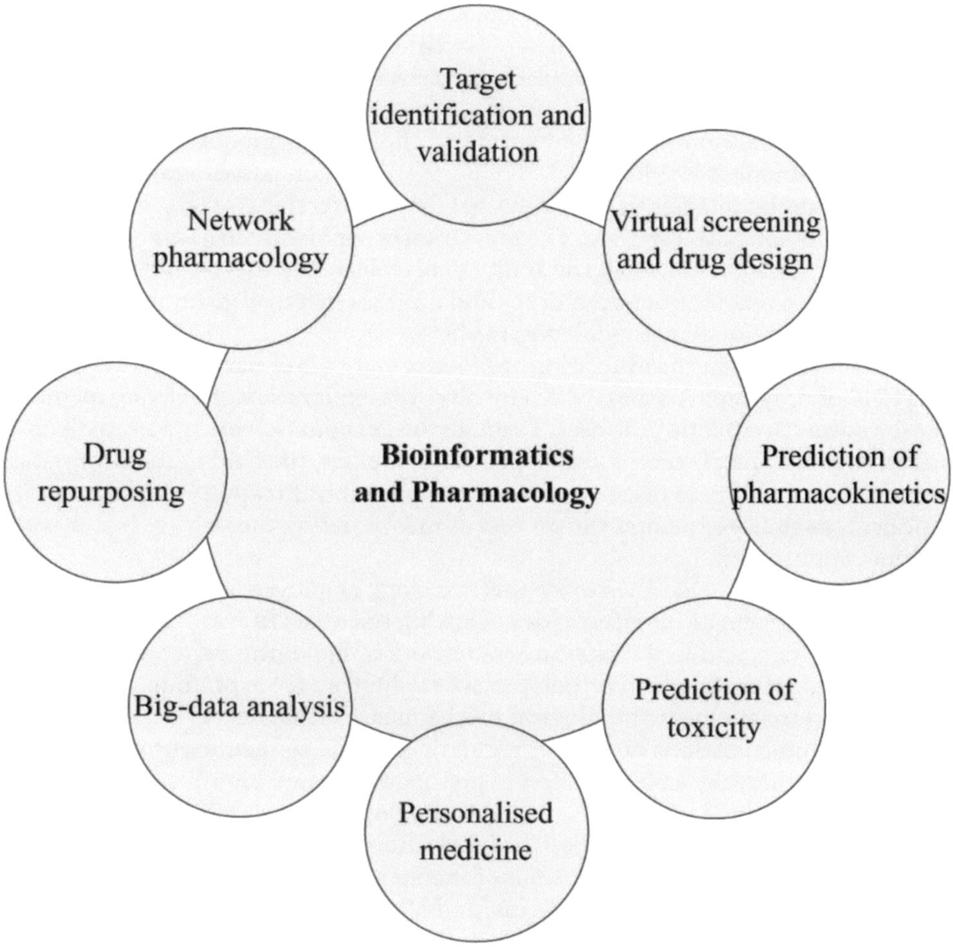

Figure 2.
Application of bioinformatics in pharmacology.

Subsequently, these targets undergo a comprehensive pharmacological validation process to verify their significance and appropriateness for therapeutic intervention.

Second, bioinformatics-driven computational techniques, such as molecular docking and molecular dynamics simulations, are utilized for the purpose of virtual screening and the generation of prospective drug candidates. This enables researchers to rapidly examine a wide range of chemical compounds, hence optimizing time and resource use throughout the initial phases of drug discovery. Bioinformatics plays a crucial role in the prioritization of candidate drugs based on their binding affinity and specificity toward target proteins through the utilization of predictive models [29, 35, 37–39]. In addition, the utilization of bioinformatics models enables the anticipation of pharmacokinetic characteristics and toxicity of potential drug candidates, encompassing absorption, distribution, metabolism, and excretion. Moreover, these models evaluate the possible toxicity and unwanted effects, assisting in the identification of safer and more efficacious medication candidates prior to their advancement into expensive experimental stages.

The merging of pharmacogenomics and bioinformatics facilitates the advancement of personalized medicine strategies. The utilization of bioinformatics enables the prediction of an individual's pharmacological response by examining their genetic composition. This data enable healthcare practitioners to customize pharmacological therapies based on the distinct genetic characteristics of individual patients, thereby enhancing therapeutic results while avoiding adverse reactions [19, 25, 40–43]. Interestingly, the vast amount of biological and clinical data produced in contemporary drug development is substantial. Bioinformatics encompasses a range of technologies and methodologies that are essential for the effective storage, management, and analysis of biological Big-Data. The utilization of sophisticated data analytics and machine learning algorithms has the ability to reveal latent patterns, biomarkers, and potential correlations between drugs and diseases that may go unnoticed when employing conventional methodologies [44].

It is noteworthy that the utilization of bioinformatics is of paramount importance in the field of drug repurposing, which involves the exploration of existing medications for novel therapeutic purposes. Through the examination of data from diverse sources, such as clinical records and molecular databases, the field of bioinformatics possesses the capability to discern innovative applications for approved pharmaceuticals. This ability expedites the process of incorporating these drugs into newer treatment approaches.

Furthermore, the field of network pharmacology employs network-based methodologies in the realm of bioinformatics, allowing scientists to examine diseases and the effects of drugs within the intricate framework of biological networks [32, 35, 45–47]. The adoption of a holistic perspective facilitates a more profound comprehension of the interrelatedness of biological mechanisms and assists in the recognition of multi-target medications capable of regulating several elements within a disease network. In essence, the amalgamation of pharmacology and bioinformatics has revolutionized the field of drug research and development, rendering it a data-centric and increasingly accurate discipline. The integration of experimental pharmacology and computational biology holds promise for enhancing drug safety and efficacy, expediting the drug development process, and ultimately enhancing patient care through personalized treatment approaches. The ongoing progress of technology will ensure that the partnership between these two fields remains a prominent aspect of pharmaceutical research and innovation.

4. Bioinformatics for toxicology and safety assessment

The field of bioinformatics plays a crucial role in the domain of toxicology and safety assessment. Bioinformatics has become an indispensable instrument in the realm of toxicology and safety assessment, facilitating the evaluation of possible dangers linked to chemical substances, medicines, and environmental factors (**Figure 3**) [48]. The below part provides the main applications of bioinformatics in the field of toxicology and safety evaluation.

The utilization of bioinformatics techniques facilitates the field of chemo-informatics, which encompasses the examination of chemical structures and their correlation with toxicity. Machine learning models that have been trained using extensive chemical databases possess the capability to forecast the toxicity of novel compounds by leveraging their structural resemblances to established dangerous substances [49]. Predictive models play a crucial role in the timely detection of potentially hazardous compounds, hence optimizing efficiency and conserving resources in the field of toxicological testing [49].

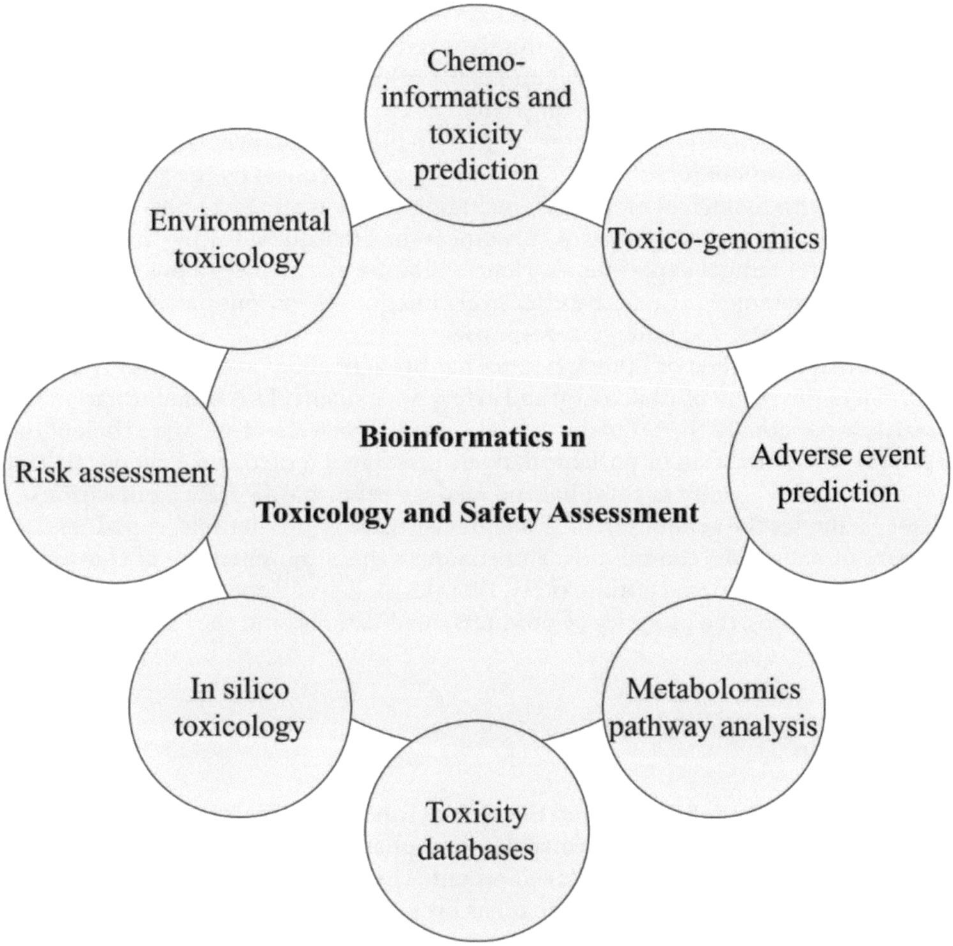

Figure 3.
Application of bioinformatics in toxicology and safety assessment.

On the other hand, toxico-genomics is an interdisciplinary field that integrates genomics and toxicology to investigate the impact of toxic chemicals on genes and gene expression. The field of bioinformatics is of utmost importance in the analysis of high-throughput gene expression data obtained from microarray and RNA sequencing investigations [50]. Through the identification of genes and pathways impacted by hazardous substances, toxicologists are able to get valuable knowledge regarding the underlying processes of toxicity, as well as prospective biomarkers that could be utilized for the early detection of such toxicity. Bioinformatics techniques are utilized to evaluate adverse event reports derived from clinical trials and post-market surveillance databases, with the aim of identifying patterns of toxicity that are linked to medications and other items. The aforementioned analyses have the potential to facilitate the discovery of safety risks that were previously unknown, hence motivating regulatory interventions or alterations in product labeling [51].

Metabolomics, a branch of bioinformatics, is dedicated to the investigation of small chemicals known as metabolites that are generated by cells and organisms. The identification of alterations in metabolite profiles resulting from toxin exposure is of paramount importance in the field of toxicology. Bioinformatics technologies are utilized for the purpose of analyzing this data and establishing connections between modifications in metabolic pathways and distinct harmful consequences [12, 52–56]. The field of in silico toxicology encompasses the application of computer simulations to forecast the toxicological characteristics of chemical substances. Bioinformatics models have the capability to predict the toxicity of a chemical by the simulation of its interactions with biological molecules, including proteins and enzymes. This methodology facilitates the prioritization of substances for subsequent testing and diminishes the necessity for animal experiments. Hence, Bioinformatics plays a pivotal role in the quantitative assessment of risks by effectively integrating various datasets pertaining to exposure, toxicity, and biological response.

In summary, the field of bioinformatics has brought about a significant transformation in the realm of toxicology and safety assessment. This transformation is primarily attributed to the provision of data-driven, cost-effective, and efficient tools that enable the evaluation of possible dangers associated with diverse chemicals and compounds. The capacity to combine and analyze extensive datasets from various sources facilitates the generation of more precise toxicity predictions, expedites the discovery of dangerous compounds, and enhances the comprehension of the underlying mechanisms associated with toxicity. Bioinformatics will continue to play a crucial role in safeguarding the integrity of products, medications, and the environment as the science progresses.

5. Conclusion

The present chapter has explored the crucial function of bioinformatics in the field of drug metabolism and pharmacology, emphasizing its importance in multiple facets of drug discovery and development. The discipline of bioinformatics has become an essential instrument that has brought about significant changes by expediting the process of identifying targets, assisting in the design of drugs based on logical principles, easing the screening of large volumes of data, and supporting the development of biomarkers for personalized medicine. Nevertheless, this process has encountered many difficulties. In order to effectively use the promise of the discipline of bioinformatics, several challenges need to be addressed, including data quality and integration, computational resources, ethical considerations, and the translation of findings into clinical applications. Notwithstanding these hurdles, the prospects for bioinformatics in the fields of drug metabolism and pharmacology appear to be auspicious. In summary, the prospects of bioinformatics in the domains of drug metabolism and pharmacology are characterized by a notable emphasis on novel advancements and cooperative efforts. As the comprehension of biological systems and computational approaches progresses, bioinformatics will persist as a pivotal catalyst in the transformation of drug development, enhancement of patient outcomes, and introduction of groundbreaking medicines to the market. Through the acknowledgment and resolution of obstacles, as well as the adoption of emerging technology, the area is positioned to experience additional significant advancements in the foreseeable future.

Author details

Dogfounianalo Somda[1], Stephen Wilson Kpordze[1,2], Mercy Jerpkorir[3], Mishell Chantelle Mahora[1], Jecinta Wanjiru Ndungu[4], Sally Wambui Kamau[4], Vera Arthur[5] and Amel Elbasyouni[1*]

1 Department of Molecular Biology and Biotechnology, Pan African University for Basic Sciences, Technology, and Innovation (PAUSTI), Kenya

2 One Health Laboratory, Spanish Laboratory Complex, University of Development Studies, Tamale, Ghana

3 Graduate School, Kenya Medical Research Institute (KEMRI), Nairobi, Kenya

4 Kenya Medical Research Institute (KEMRI), Nairobi, Kenya

5 Department of Biotechnology, Fort Valley State University, USA

*Address all correspondence to: elbasyouni.amel@students.jkuat.ac.ke; elbasyouni.amel@hotmail.com

References

[1] Yildirim O, Gottwald M, Schüler P, Michel MC. Opportunities and challenges for drug development: Public–private partnerships, adaptive designs and big data. Frontiers in Pharmacology [Internet]. 2016;7:761. Available from: http://journal.frontiersin.org/article/10.3389/fphar.2016.00461/full

[2] Villoutreix BO. Post-pandemic drug discovery and development: Facing present and future challenges. Frontiers in Drug Discovery. 2021;**1**:728469

[3] Schenone M, Dančík V, Wagner BK, Clemons PA. Target identification and mechanism of action in chemical biology and drug discovery. Nature Chemical Biology. 2013;**9**(4):232-240

[4] Ma H, Zhao H. Drug target inference through pathway analysis of genomics data. Advanced Drug Delivery Reviews. 2013;**65**(7):966-972

[5] Emmerich CH, Gamboa LM, Hofmann MCJ, Bonin-Andresen M, Arbach O, Schendel P, et al. Improving target assessment in biomedical research: The GOT-IT recommendations. Nature Reviews. Drug Discovery. 2021;**20**(1):64-81

[6] Cava C, Bertoli G, Castiglioni I. In silico identification of drug target pathways in breast cancer subtypes using pathway cross-talk inhibition. Journal of Translational Medicine. 2018;**16**(1):154

[7] Steinmetz KL, Spack EG. The basics of preclinical drug development for neurodegenerative disease indications. BMC Neurology. 2009;**9**(Suppl 1):S2

[8] Singh N, Vayer P, Tanwar S, Poyet JL, Tsaioun K, Villoutreix BO. Drug discovery and development: Introduction to the general public and patient groups. Frontiers in Drug Discovery. 2023;**3**:1201419

[9] Mohs RC, Greig NH. Drug discovery and development: Role of basic biological research. Alzheimer's & Dementia: Translational Research & Clinical Interventions. 2017;**3**(4):651-657

[10] Singh S, Loke YK. Drug safety assessment in clinical trials: Methodological challenges and opportunities. Trials. 2012;**13**(1):138

[11] Weaver RJ, Valentin JP. Today's challenges to de-risk and predict drug safety in human "mind-the-gap". Toxicological Sciences. 2019;**167**(2):307-321

[12] Bioinformatics XX, Discovery D. Current Topics in Medicinal Chemistry. 2017;**17**(15):1709-1726

[13] Wishart DS. Bioinformatics in drug development and assessment. Drug Metabolism Reviews. 2005;**37**(2):279-310

[14] Sankar A, Ranu S, Raman K. Predicting novel metabolic pathways through subgraph mining. Bioinformatics. 2017;**33**(24):3955-3963

[15] Baranwal M, Magner A, Elvati P, Saldinger J, Violi A, Hero AO. A deep learning architecture for metabolic pathway prediction. Bioinformatics. 2020;**36**(8):2547-2553

[16] Shah HA, Liu J, Yang Z, Feng J. Review of machine learning methods for the prediction and reconstruction of metabolic pathways. Frontiers in Molecular Biosciences. 2021;**8**:634141

[17] Wang P, Schumacher AM, Shiu SH. Computational prediction of plant metabolic pathways. Current Opinion in Plant Biology. 2022;**66**:102171

[18] Hamdalla MA, Rajasekaran S, Grant DF, Măndoiu II. Metabolic pathway predictions for metabolomics: A molecular structure matching approach. Journal of Chemical Information and Modeling. 2015;**55**(3):709-718

[19] Wooller SK, Benstead-Hume G, Chen X, Ali Y, Pearl FMG. Bioinformatics in translational drug discovery. Bioscience Reports. 2017;**37**(4):BSR20160180

[20] Huang LC, Wu X, Chen JY. Predicting adverse side effects of drugs. BMC Genomics. 2011;**12**(S5):S11

[21] Liang X, Fu Y, Qu L, Zhang P, Chen Y. Prediction of drug side effects with transductive matrix co-completion. Bioinformatics. 2023;**39**(1):btad006

[22] Yamanishi Y, Pauwels E, Kotera M. Drug side-effect prediction based on the integration of chemical and biological spaces. Journal of Chemical Information and Modeling. 2012;**52**(12):3284-3292

[23] Chen Y, Juan L, Lv X, Shi L. Bioinformatics research on drug sensitivity prediction. Frontiers in Pharmacology. 2021;**12**:799712

[24] Wu Z, Peng Y, Yu Z, Li W, Liu G, Tang Y. NetInfer: A web server for prediction of targets and therapeutic and adverse effects via network-based inference methods. Journal of Chemical Information and Modeling. 2020;**60**(8):3687-3691

[25] Katara P. Role of bioinformatics and pharmacogenomics in drug discovery and development process. Network Modeling Analysis in Health Informatics and Bioinformatics. 2013;**2**(4):225-230

[26] Saberian N, Peyvandipour A, Donato M, Ansari S, Draghici S. A new computational drug repurposing method using established disease–drug pair knowledge. Bioinformatics. 2019;**35**(19):3672-3678

[27] Tanoli Z, Seemab U, Scherer A, Wennerberg K, Tang J, Vähä-Koskela M. Exploration of databases and methods supporting drug repurposing: A comprehensive survey. Briefings in Bioinformatics. 2021;**22**(2):1656-1678

[28] Amiri Souri E, Chenoweth A, Karagiannis SN, Tsoka S. Drug repurposing and prediction of multiple interaction types via graph embedding. BMC Bioinformatics. 2023;**24**(1):202

[29] Duarte Y, Márquez-Miranda V, Miossec MJ, González-Nilo F. Integration of target discovery, drug discovery and drug delivery: A review on computational strategies. WIREs Nanomedicine Nanobiotechnology. 2019;**11**(4):e1554

[30] Ma R. Bioinformatics-key to drug discovery and development. Journal of Pharmaceutical Research. 2017;**1**(5):000126

[31] Berger SI, Iyengar R. Network analyses in systems pharmacology. Bioinformatics. 2009;**25**(19):2466-2472

[32] Leung EL, Cao ZW, Jiang ZH, Zhou H, Liu L. Network-based drug discovery by integrating systems biology and computational technologies. Briefings in Bioinformatics. 2013;**14**(4):491-505

[33] Alam MS, Sultana A, MDS R, Amanullah M, Kabir SR, MDNH M. Integrated bioinformatics and statistical approaches to explore molecular biomarkers for breast cancer diagnosis,

prognosis and therapies. PLoS One. 2022;**17**(5):e0268967

[34] Hermawan A, Putri H. Bioinformatics analysis reveals the potential target of rosiglitazone as an antiangiogenic agent for breast cancer therapy. BMC Genomic Data. 2022;**23**(1):72

[35] Elbasyouni A, Wilson Kpordze S, Suliman Hussein H, Soro O, Mulondo S, Nshimirimana J, et al. The crosstalk between phytotherapy and bioinformatics in the management of cancer. In: Recent Advances in Alternative Medicine [Working Title] [Internet]. London, UK: IntechOpen; 2023. Available from: https://www.intechopen.com/online-first/1141766

[36] Ren Y, Deng R, Zhang Q, Li J, Han B, Ye P. Bioinformatics analysis of key genes in triple negative breast cancer and validation of oncogene PLK1. Annals of Translational Medicine. 2020;**8**(24):1637-1637

[37] Santos LHS, Ferreira RS, Caffarena ER. Integrating molecular docking and molecular dynamics simulations. In: De Azevedo WF, editor. Docking Screens for Drug Discovery [Internet]. New York, NY: Springer New York; 2019. pp. 13-34. (Methods in Molecular Biology; vol. 2053). Available from: http://link.springer.com/10.1007/978-1-4939-9752-7_2

[38] Subhaswaraj P, Siddhardha B. Molecular docking and molecular dynamic simulation approaches for drug development and repurposing of drugs for severe acute respiratory syndrome-Coronavirus-2. In: Computational Approaches for Novel Therapeutic and Diagnostic Designing to Mitigate SARS-CoV-2 Infection [Internet]. Elsevier; 2022. pp. 207-246. Available from: https://linkinghub.elsevier.com/retrieve/pii/B9780323911726000078

[39] Vidal-Limon A, Aguilar-Toalá JE, Liceaga AM. Integration of molecular docking analysis and molecular dynamics simulations for studying food proteins and bioactive peptides. Journal of Agricultural and Food Chemistry. 2022;**70**(4):934-943

[40] Fernald GH, Capriotti E, Daneshjou R, Karczewski KJ, Altman RB. Bioinformatics challenges for personalized medicine. Bioinformatics. 2011;**27**(13):1741-1748

[41] Li YY, Jones SJ. Drug repositioning for personalized medicine. Genome Medicine. 2012;**4**(3):27

[42] Hartl D, De Luca V, Kostikova A, Laramie J, Kennedy S, Ferrero E, et al. Translational precision medicine: An industry perspective. Journal of Translational Medicine. 2021;**19**(1):245

[43] Stern AM, Schurdak ME, Bahar I, Berg JM, Taylor DL. A perspective on implementing a quantitative systems pharmacology platform for drug discovery and the advancement of personalized medicine. SLAS Discovery. 2016;**21**(6):521-534

[44] Mak KK, Pichika MR. Artificial intelligence in drug development: Present status and future prospects. Drug Discovery Today. 2019;**24**(3):773-780

[45] Batool S, Javed MR, Aslam S, Noor F, Javed HMF, Seemab R, et al. Network pharmacology and bioinformatics approach reveals the multi-target pharmacological mechanism of Fumaria indica in the treatment of liver cancer. Pharmaceuticals. 2022;**15**(6):654

[46] Li L, Wang X, Guo X, Li Y, Song Q, Li A. Network pharmacology and

computer-aided drug design to explored potential targets of Lianhua Qingwen and Qingfei Paidu decoction for COVID-19. Frontiers in Pharmacology. 2022;**13**:1013428

[47] Jin J, Chen B, Zhan X, Zhou Z, Liu H, Dong Y. Network pharmacology and molecular docking study on the mechanism of colorectal cancer treatment using Xiao-chai-Hu-Tang. PLoS One. 2021;**16**(6):e0252508

[48] Afshari CA, Hamadeh HK, Bushel PR. The evolution of bioinformatics in toxicology: Advancing toxicogenomics. Toxicological Sciences. 2011;**120**(Suppl 1):S225-S237

[49] Pognan F. The evolving role of investigative toxicology in the pharmaceutical industry. Nature Reviews. Drug Discovery. 2023;**22**:317-335

[50] Singh AV. Integrative toxicogenomics: Advancing precision medicine and toxicology through artificial intelligence and OMICs technology. Biomedicine & Pharmacotherapy. 2023;**163**:114784

[51] Yamagata Y, Yamada H, Horii I. Current status and future perspective of computational toxicology in drug safety assessment under ontological intellection. Journal of Toxicological Sciences. 2019;**44**(11):721-735. DOI: 10.2131/jts.44.721. PMID: 31708530

[52] Palermo A. Metabolomics- and systems-biology-guided discovery of metabolite lead compounds and druggable targets. Drug Discovery Today. 2023;**28**(2):103460

[53] Barupal DK, Fan S, Fiehn O. Integrating bioinformatics approaches for a comprehensive interpretation of metabolomics datasets. Current Opinion in Biotechnology. 2019;**54**:1-9

[54] Alarcon-Barrera JC. Recent advances in metabolomics analysis for early drug development. Drug Discovery Today. 2022;**27**(6):1763-1773

[55] Paananen J, Fortino V. An omics perspective on drug target discovery platforms. Briefings in Bioinformatics. 2020;**21**(6):1937-1953

[56] Phapale P. Pharmaco-metabolomics opportunities in drug development and clinical research. Analytical Science Advances. 2021;**2**:611-616

Section 3

Drug Metabolism and Bioanalysis

Chapter 6

The Modification Strategies for Enhancing the Metabolic Stabilities and Pharmacokinetics of Aptamer Drug Candidates

Yuan Ma, Yihao Zhang, Zefeng Chen, Yuan Tian and Ge Zhang

Abstract

Aptamers are single-stranded DNA or RNA that can mimic the functional properties of monoclonal antibodies. Aptamers have high affinity and specificity for their target molecules, which can make them a promising alternative to therapeutic antibodies or peptide ligands. However, many aptamer drug candidates in clinical development have been discontinued due to suboptimal metabolic stabilities and pharmacokinetics. To address these issues, chemical modification can be used to enhance the metabolic stability and prolong the half-life of aptamer candidates. The chapter reviewed published data regarding the metabolic stability and pharmacokinetics of aptamer drug candidates from preclinical and clinical studies. The benefits and possible shortcomings of current modification strategies used in these aptamers were briefly discussed.

Keywords: metabolic stability, pharmacokinetics, aptamer, chemical modification, renal clearance

1. Introduction

Aptamers are single-stranded DNA or RNA oligonucleotide-based synthetic molecules that can replicate the functional features of monoclonal antibodies. Nucleic acid aptamers are generally screened from a library of random nucleic acids utilizing systematic evolution of ligands by exponential enrichment (SELEX) technology [1]. To effectively create an aptamer against a given target molecule, the SELEX procedure requires multiple phases. The aptamer and desired target molecule are incubated to initiate the binding affinity process, which is followed by the division of bound and unbound sequences. After that, binding sequences are amplified by PCR, and ssDNA is extracted to start a new cycle [2, 3]. As a result, aptamers have a high affinity and selectivity for a wide range of target molecules, including peptides, proteins, tiny compounds, and even living cells. Because inhibitory aptamers that affect the activity of pathogenic target proteins may be utilized as therapeutic agents directly, they are a viable alternative to therapeutic antibodies or peptide ligands [4]. Aptamers

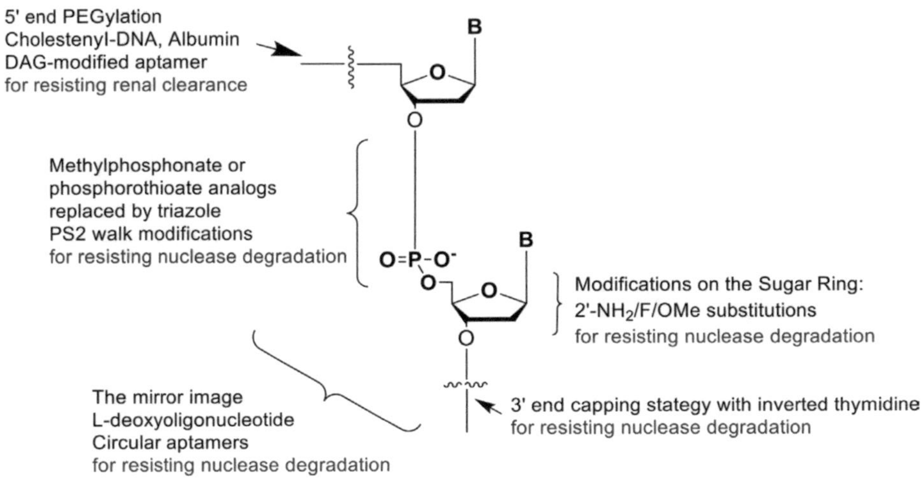

Figure 1.
The common strategies in the chemical modifications of nucleic acid aptamers and their purposes.

have several benefits over antibodies, including ease of synthesis, reduced time and cost, lesser immunogenicity, greater stability, and superior refold ability. As a result, aptamers are prospective replacements for homologous antibodies. The United States Food and Drug Administration (FDA) granted approval for the initial aptamer drug (Macugen®) to treat wet-form neovascular age-related macular degeneration (AMD) in 2004 [5, 6]. Several therapeutic aptamers are currently undergoing clinical trials in phases II and III.

However, aptamer candidates' druggability can be considerably impacted by their metabolic stability and pharmacokinetics. Indeed, due to inadequate qualities in these domains, certain aptamers under clinical development have been abandoned. The renal filtration cut-off value is 30–50 kDa. Native nucleic acid aptamers face challenges *in vivo* due to their susceptibility to nuclease-mediated cleavage and rapid renal filtration, primarily attributed to the abundance of serum nucleases and their relatively low molecular weight (20 kDa). Consequently, these aptamers are rapidly eliminated from the body, leading to a short biological half-life. These are key issues that are impeding the clinical translation of the nucleic acid aptamer. Chemical modification can be utilized to improve the metabolic stability and half-life of aptamer candidates to solve these difficulties. To begin, changes in metabolic stability may increase nucleic acid aptamer formation while increasing nuclease resistance. Second, long-term alterations might permit nucleic acid aptamer boosting molecular weight substantially over the renal filtration cut-off level (**Figure 1**). The chapter reviewed published data regarding the metabolic stability and pharmacokinetics of aptamer drug candidates from preclinical and clinical studies. The advantages and disadvantages of current modification procedures employed in these aptamers were briefly explored.

2. Strategies for enhancing metabolic stability of aptamers

Modification tactics for improving metabolic stability of aptamer drug candidates may be carried out in two ways: pre-SELEX chemical modifications and post-SELEX chemical modifications. Pre-SELEX alterations mostly entail chemical changes that are critical for the aptamer's functions [6]. Nucleobase modifications and genetic alphabet extension are typical examples. The goal of adding these new chemical moieties or bases to aptamers is to improve their functionality and allow them to engage with additional targets. These changes immediately affect the three-dimensional structure of aptamers [7]. Aptamer activity may be fully eliminated by adding these chemical groups following SELEX. As a result, pre-SELEX alteration is the most effective strategy to minimize activity loss. The fundamental disadvantage of this method is that the alteration might impair the nucleotide's capacity to act as a substrate for DNA or RNA polymerase [8]. During solid-phase chemical synthesis, changes at multiple sites are added to preselected aptamers in post-SELEX techniques for the best performances such as high affinity, high stability, and high specificity. Because aptamer affinity/specificity and function are structure-dependent, post-SELEX alteration may modify the intrinsic characteristics and folding structures of the original aptamers, compromising binding affinity [9]. As a result, alterations must be properly tailored to the intended functions [10]. Unfortunately, general guidelines do not exist for all aptamers, and tedious evaluation/optimization is frequently required [11]. The following are some of the most prevalent nucleic acid aptamer modifications:

2.1 Nucleobases modifications

The research on SELEX using unnatural nucleobases has seen rapid growth in recent years, with two main categories of efforts: (1) creating unnatural base pair systems that are independent of Watson-Crick base pairs and (2) integrating peptide-like functional groups into native nucleobases [12]. However, a significant challenge in using unnatural nucleobases in SELEX is the need for encoding and decoding these nucleotides throughout the selection process, which often requires compatibility with polymerases. Ensuring high accuracy in base pairing selection with or between modified bases during the encoding and decoding stages is another obstacle in nucleobase modifications. To overcome these challenges and expand the range of nucleobase changes available for in vitro aptamer selection, researchers have developed several innovative strategies.

2.2 Ribose modifications

The creation of medicinal antisense oligonucleotides spurred early advances in chemical modifications of aptamers. These changes were made largely to improve resistance to nuclease-mediated degradation [13]. Initially, changes were introduced at the 2′-position of the ribose sugar unit. Modifications at all nucleotides, on the other hand, are seldom tolerated since a sugar alteration reduces aptamer activity [14]. Point-by-point changes and activity testing take time and money. As a result, including changed nucleotides in the SELEX procedure should be investigated. The presence of a polymerase that can be modified is the most significant aspect. Nowadays, replacing fluorine (2′-F) (**Figure 2a**), methoxy (2′-OMe) (**Figure 2b**), or amino (2′-NH_2) (**Figure 2c**) groups for the 2′-hydroxy residue of RNA greatly improves aptamer stability against nuclease degradation [15].

2′-Aminopyrimidines were utilized in the first ribose-modified SELEX experiment [16]. Then, a change was made to the T7 RNA polymerase to improve substrate compatibility. It has been demonstrated that 2′-fluoro and 2′-deoxypyrimidine are

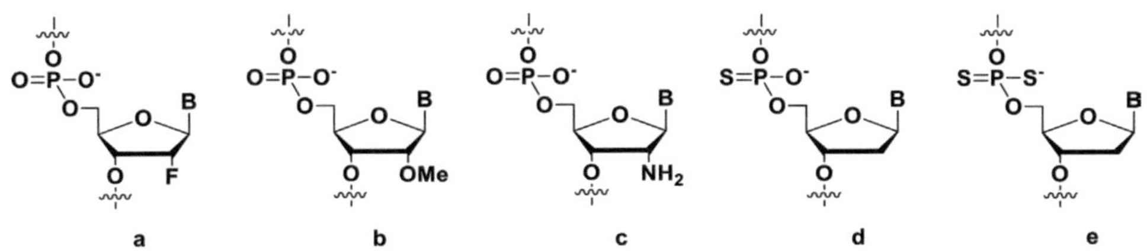

Figure 2.
Chemical structures of modifications for the improvement of nuclease resistance of aptamers: (a) 2′-fluoro-RNA (2′-F); (b) 2′-methoxy-RNA (2′-OMe); (c) 2′-amino-RNA (2′-NH2); (d) Thiophosphorus-DNA/RNA; (e) Phosphorothioate-DNA/RNA.

incorporated by T7 RNA polymerase with the Y639F mutation [17–19]. Pyrimidine alterations have frequently been used as a starting point for aptamer synthesis because they prevent RNase A-mediated degradation [5]. However, in contrast to 2′-fluoropyrimidine, 2′-aminopyrimidine is seldom used in the present SELEX technique due to reduced coupling efficiencies in chemical synthesis, a predilection for the C2′-endo ribose conformation, and a detrimental influence on base pairing stability [20].

Pegaptanib (Macugen®), the sole FDA-approved oligonucleotide-based medicine on the market, exemplifies a sugar-modified aptamer. It was developed *in vitro* using a combination of unmodified purine nucleotides and 2′-F-pyrimidine nucleotides [9]. The remaining unmodified purine nucleotides were converted to 2′-OMe units through solid-phase synthesis. Additionally, two 2'-F-modified thrombin-binding aptamers (PG13 and PG14) showed a fourfold increase in thrombin-binding affinity and up to a sevenfold improvement in nuclease resistance. In 10% FBS, the improved aptamer's G-quadruplex stability was enhanced up to 48-fold [21]. Lin et al. created a human neutrophil elastase (HNE) aptamer with a 2'-NH2 group, demonstrating high binding affinity and 10-fold increased stability in human serum and urine compared to the original aptamer [22]. It has also been found that basic fibroblast growth factor (bFGF) can be effectively inhibited by RNA ligands modified with 2′-amino-2′-deoxypyrimidine. When incubated in human serum, 2′-aminopyrimidine-modified RNA aptamers are much more stable than naturally unmodified RNA aptamers (>1000-folds) [23]. In another study by Green et al., Vascular permeability factor/vascular endothelial growth factor (VPF/VEGF)-binding RNA and DNA aptamers demonstrated a good binding affinity and nuclease resistance [24].

2.3 Phosphate modifications

Modifications to the phosphate portion of aptamer are thought to be a significant technique for aiding aptamer's resistance to nuclease *in vivo*. Sulfur can replace two nonbridging oxygens to generate thiophosphorus (PS) (**Figure 2d**) and phosphorodithioate (PS2) (**Figure 2e**). Solid-phase synthesis had developed PS-modified DNA. The vulcanization phase replaces the oxidation step in the PS DNA synthesis. Beaucage reagent is used for vulcanizing a recently generated phosphite triester ester. Two isomers would be produced as a result of this reaction [25]. Through high-performance liquid chromatography (HPLC), a single PS modification can be isolated, and synthetic methods can produce several pure diastereomers of PS modifications [26]. The PS modification's ability to enhance the affinity between aptamers and targets can be illustrated with the following examples.

Wu et al. created two DNA aptamers, XQ-2 and a shortened variant termed XQ-2d, to target Pancreatic Ductal Adenocarcinoma (PDAC), the most frequent pancreatic adenocarcinoma [27]. They made phosphorothioate and 2'-OMe derivatives of XQ-2d to boost serum stability; however, they discovered that the thioaptamer form of XQ-2d had decreased binding to PL45 cells, while the 2'-OMe version did not [28]. Chen et al. investigated a 50-polyethylene glycol (PEG)-modified form of Adipo8 with phosphonothioate linkages placed right after the first base and just before the last base [29]. When examined in tissue culture and *in vivo*, the addition of these two thioate connections boosted serum stability by a tiny but statistically significant amount. Because this aptamer can identify white adipocytes from brown adipocytes and preadipocytes, it might be used to provide adipocyte-specific treatment [30]. PS2 alterations, which replace both nonbridging oxygen atoms with sulfur, have been incorporated into RNA aptamers chosen for binding to VEGF165. PS2 alterations increase nuclease resistance and aptamer stability in human serum [31].

2.4 Isomerized nucleoside modifications

2.4.1 Spiegelmers

A method for altering aptamers is the creation of "mirror-image" aptamers, also known as spiegelmers (**Figure 3a**). Spiegelmers counteract nucleases' stereoselectivity by inverting the chirality centers inside sugar molecules, resulting in a mirror image of wild-type DNA or RNA. This structural change makes spiegelmers more stable *in vivo*, as they evade recognition by nucleases and the immune system [32]. Traditionally, spiegelmer selection involved a two-step process, where researchers first created a mirror-imaged target and selected D-aptamers using standard SELEX. The chosen D-aptamer was then converted into the corresponding spiegelmer [33]. However, recent advancements in molecular systems capable of replicating and transcribing L-nucleotides have simplified and reduced the cost of the selection process [34].

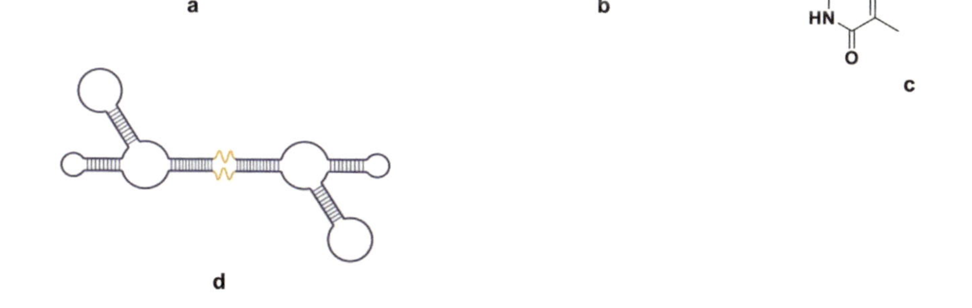

Figure 3.
Chemical structures of second-generation modifications for the improvement of nuclease resistance of aptamers: (a) Spiegelmers; (b) d–/l-isonucleoside; (c) inverted thymidine; (d) circular Aptamers.

Spiegelmers have found applications in cancer research and therapy. For example, Roccaro et al. developed a spiegelmer targeting SDF-1 to inhibit bone marrow metastasis of multiple myeloma cells [35]. In cell and animal tests, the spiegelmer effectively neutralized SDF-1, demonstrating its potential to inhibit metastasis. NOX-A12, an SDF-1 binding spiegelmer, is currently undergoing phase II clinical trials, showing an 86% response rate against relapsed/refractory chronic lymphocytic leukemia. However, further research is needed before NOX-A12 can be approved as a therapeutically viable drug [33].

2.4.2 d–/l-Isonucleoside modifications

Isonucleosides are nucleoside analogs where the bases are repositioned to the nucleoside's 2′ or 3′ position (**Figure 3b**). Oligonucleotides incorporating isonucleosides exhibit increased resistance to nuclease-mediated hydrolysis [36]. Yang et al. explored the potential of d–/l-isonucleosides as modifiers for three aptamers (TBA, GBI-10, and AS1411). The strategic incorporation of d–/l-isonucleosides, particularly in the loop regions, led to notable enhancements in spatial conformation stability and chemical robustness within the modified aptamers [37, 38]. Consequently, the modified aptamers exhibited significantly heightened resistance against biodegradation. Interestingly, modifications with L-isonucleosides had a more profound impact on enhancing the biological activity of the aptamers compared to changes with D-isonucleosides. These findings underscore the significance of isonucleoside chirality in influencing the functional characteristics of modified aptamers.

2.4.3 Inverted nucleoside modifications

Oligodeoxynucleotides were commonly modified with inverted thymidine (5′-,3′-inverted T) (**Figure 3c**) to render them resistant to nucleases. Pegaptanib also has a 40 kDa poly (ethylene glycol) moiety at the 5′ end to help with renal clearance, as well as a 3′-3′-linked deoxythymidine residue to help with nuclease destruction. Despite these changes, pegaptanib retained an exceedingly high affinity for its VEGF165 target and demonstrated sustained in vitro [39] stability. Moreover, the antifactor IXa RNA aptamer RB06 is composed of unmodified purine nucleosides, 2′-F-pyrimidine nucleosides, 5′-terminal 40 kDa-PEG moiety, and 3′-terminal 3′-inverted deoxythymidine preserved excellent affinity to the target, high in vivo stability and robust anticoagulant efficacy [40].

2.5 Nuclease-resistant circular Aptamers

The creation of circular aptamers (**Figure 3d**), which solve the difficulty of metabolic instability, is a recent accomplishment in aptamer modification. Aptamers can avoid exonuclease degradation by connecting the 5′ and 3′ termini of nucleic acids to create a closed circular shape, resulting in increased resistance to nucleases [40]. King et al. created multivalent circular aptamers with anticoagulant activity, illustrating the power of cyclization in the creation of functional aptamers [41]. Cyclization enhances aptamer resistance to nucleases, increasing heat stability and guaranteeing structural homogeneity. Tan et al. reported the development of bivalent circular aptamers employing three aptamers that target live cancer cells (Sgc8, TD05, and XQ-2d) [42–44]. The cyclization technique provides an economical and practical approach to improving the stability and binding ability of aptamers, allowing them to be used in diagnostic and therapy. The usage of circular aptamers is a viable option for increasing aptamer stability and functional qualities, bringing up new possibilities for their use in a variety of biological applications [45].

3. Strategies for prolonging the half-life of aptamers

Due to their quick elimination via renal filtration, tiny aptamers continue to provide a barrier for renal clearance (**Figure 4**). To solve this, several techniques, including the attachment of cholesterol, PEG, proteins, liposomes, and other materials, have been reported. PEGylation, in particular, is a well-established and commonly utilized technique for prolonging medication half-life. Other approaches, such as lipid nanoparticle delivery systems and attachment to bioactive natural proteins, have also been used to improve the metabolic stability and pharmacokinetic features of therapeutic nucleic acid aptamers. Alternative PEGylation approaches, such as employing long-half-life proteins and low molecular weight coupling agents, have also been investigated to extend the half-life of aptamers. These methodologies may be adapted

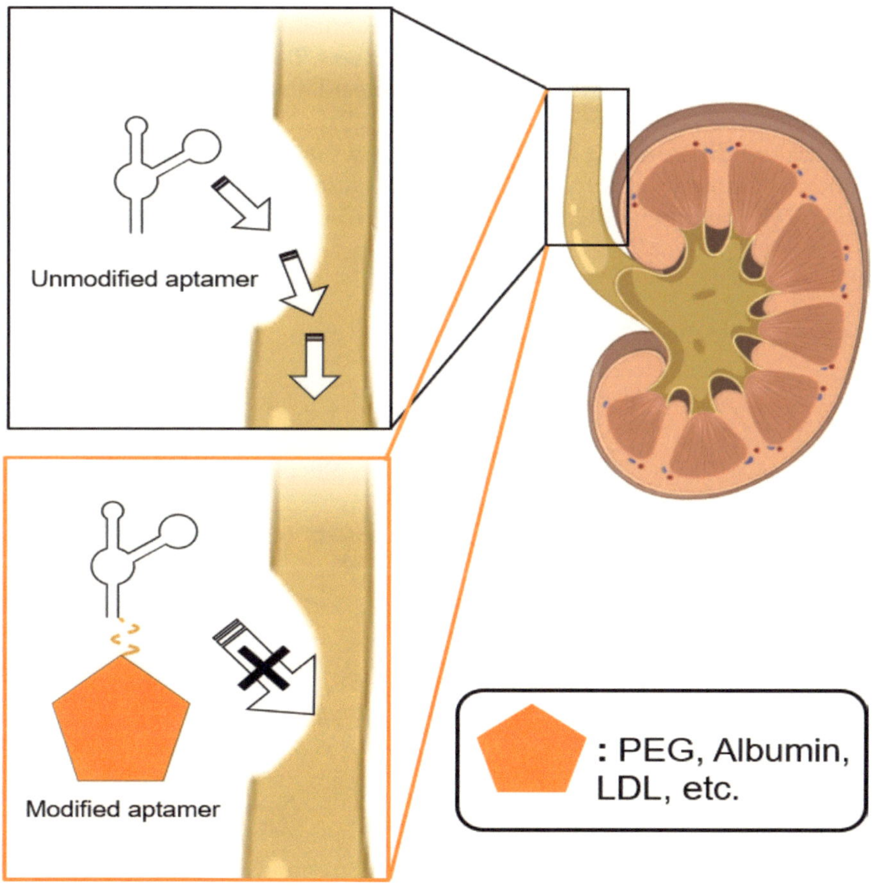

Figure 4.
Schematic illustration of chemical modification prevents the aptamer from renal clearance.

to specific aptamer applications and therapeutic purposes, allowing for the creation of aptamers with increased stability, bioavailability, and circulation half-life.

3.1 Polyethylene glycol

Polyethylene glycol (PEG) (**Figure 5a**) is a group of synthetic polymers with high molecular weight, having linear or branched structures and hydroxyl groups [46]. Its molecular weight can vary from a few hundred to tens of thousands, leading to diverse physicochemical characteristics. PEG with a molecular weight below 700 remains liquid at typical temperatures, while PEG exceeding 1000 assumes a predominantly solid form [47]. Thanks to its low toxicity and immunogenicity, the FDA has granted approval for PEG's pharmaceutical applications. PEGs weighing less than 30 kDa are typically cleared through the kidneys, while those with molecular weights exceeding 20 kDa are excreted in feces [48].

The process of PEGylation involves attaching PEG to macromolecules like proteins, peptides, and nucleic acids. This coating of medication molecules with a hydrophilic shield diminishes immune recognition and enzymatic degradation within the body [49]. Additionally, PEGylation augments the size of drug molecules, thereby reducing renal clearance, as it predominantly relies on the molecule's size. Consequently, PEGylated drugs often exhibit increased efficacy due to their prolonged biological half-life. Several examples highlight how PEGylation effectively extends the biological half-life of medicinal aptamers. The biological half-life of aptamers is extended differently by different molecular weights of PEG. To reduce renal clearance, the initial version of the von Willebrand factor (VWF) aptamer ARC1779 was modified with a 20 kDa-PEG moiety. However, its limited half-life of approximately 2 hours restricted its clinical application [50]. In contrast, the second-generation VWF aptamer ARC15105 was developed with higher molecular weight

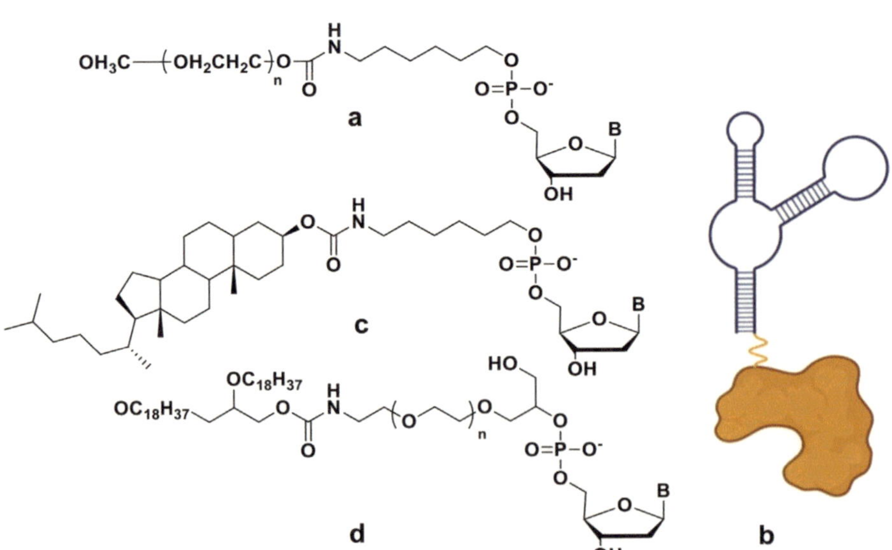

Figure 5.
Chemical structures of modifications for prolonging the half-life of aptamers. (a) Cholesterol-oligonucleotide conjugates; (b) polyethylene glycol (PEG)-oligonucleotide conjugates; (c) dialkylglycerol (DAG)-oligonucleotide conjugates; (d) albumin-oligonucleotide conjugates.

PEG moieties (40 kDa), leading to a significantly extended half-life of 66 hours while maintaining the same level of VWF inhibition [51].

Pegaptanib, commercialized as Macugen, is the first FDA-approved PEGylated RNA aptamer for the treatment of age-related macular degeneration. Pegaptanib binds to vascular endothelial growth factor (VEGF) selectively and inhibits its interaction with VEGF receptors, hence reducing neoangiogenesis. Pegaptanib has been modified with a PEG moiety of 40 kDa. Pegaptanib exhibited a half-life of around ten days in clinical studies, and therapy with pegaptanib maintained steady visual acuity in a substantial percentage of patients [52]. NOX-A12, also known as Olaptesed pegol, is an RNA Spiegelmer modified with a 40 kDa branched PEG moiety [53]. It selectively binds to the chemokine CXCL12, hindering its interaction with CXCR4 and CXCR7. This inhibition effectively hampers angiogenesis and metastasis, thereby enhancing cancer treatment. In phase I/II clinical trial, NOX-A12 demonstrated a half-life of 53.2 hours at a dose of 4 mg/kg. Similarly, another PEGylated RNA Spiegelmer, NOX-H94 or lexapeptid pegol, exhibits preferential binding to human hepcidin, leading to the inactivation of its biological function and simultaneously improving blood iron content and transferrin saturation. NOX-H94 was also modified with a 40 kDa branched PEG moiety. It displayed a dose-dependent increase in serum iron content and transferrin saturation, with a half-life ranging from 14.1 to 26.1 hours [54]. These findings illustrate the potential of PEGylated RNA Spiegelmers as promising candidates in various therapeutic applications.

While PEGylation has been frequently used to extend the biological half-life of liposomes for drug administration, repeated injections of PEGylated liposomes can cause an accelerated blood clearance (ABC) phenomenon, shortening the biological half-life. Aside from PEGylation, several methods for prolonging the half-life of nucleic acid aptamers have been investigated, including PAS [55] (proline, alanine, and serine sequences) and PLGA [56] (poly(lactic-*co*-glycolic acid)). PASylation is accomplished by the use of synthetic polypeptides composed of Pro, Ala, and/or Ser amino acids, which have characteristics similar to PEG. The synthetic polymer PLGA, which is made of lactic acid and glycolic acid, has low toxicity, biodegradability, and biocompatibility. PLGA has been used in nanocarriers for medication delivery systems, including nucleic acid delivery systems. PEGylation has long been the primary approach for increasing medication half-life. However, due to the mixed nature of commercial reagents, their usage has prompted concerns about the consistency of PEGylated medicinal products, as well as safety and bioaccumulation difficulties [57]. Hypersensitivity responses and the development of antibodies against PEG can result in decreased effectiveness in prolonging biological half-life [58]. As a result, various PEGylation techniques have been investigated in order to increase the half-life of biopharmaceuticals. Furthermore, connecting nucleic acid aptamers to bioactive natural proteins is a promising technique with future development potential.

3.2 Albumin

Human serum albumin (HSA) (**Figure 5b**) is a common protein in human plasma with a high affinity for drug binding (approximately 40 mg/mL). Utilizing its long biological half-life of around 19 days [59] and a molecular weight of 67 kDa, albumin has become increasingly popular as a drug carrier in pharmaceutical applications [60]. Extending the half-life of aptamers can be achieved by improving the blood circulation half-life of HSA through its interaction with the neonatal Fc receptor (FcRn), which facilitates cellular recycling [61]. This approach can enhance the stability and persistence of aptamers in the bloodstream, ultimately leading to improved therapeutic efficacy. Creating albumin-aptamer conjugates through chemical conjugation of aptamers with albumin is a favored method for aptamer administration.

A novel albumin-oligodeoxynucleotide assembly method was developed by Matthias Kuhlmann et al., involving the conjugation of albumin's cysteine residue at position 34 (cys34) with maleimide-derivatized oligodeoxynucleotides at the 3′ or 5′ end [62]. This construct remained stable in 10% serum over a 24-hour period. Similarly, Julie Schmkel et al. devised a site-specific conjugation technique for attaching an anticoagulant aptamer to recombinant albumins, ensuring the retention of aptamer activity and albumin receptor engagement [63]. Remarkably, the binding affinity of the aptamer conjugate to FcRn was significantly strengthened when it was coupled to recombinant albumin engineered to have enhanced FcRn affinity. These innovative techniques have the potential to significantly alter the pharmacokinetic profile of aptamers, paving the way for improved therapeutic outcomes. Apart from albumin, the human immunoglobulin G (IgG) Fc domain is another long-half-life protein in human blood that can be employed to modify aptamers and enhance their pharmacokinetic characteristics. The IgG Fc domain is commonly utilized to improve the pharmacokinetics of biologically active proteins or peptides [64]. *In vivo*, IgG exhibits a longer half-life compared to albumin. Therefore, when a drug is conjugated with the Fc domain of IgG, it displays superior pharmacokinetic properties compared to albumin-based conjugates. This modification strategy holds promise for extending the circulation time of aptamers and enhancing their therapeutic efficacy. Furthermore, the Fc domain has a molecular weight equivalent to albumin or PEG. Although no study has been published on using the Fc domain to conjugate aptamers for half-life extension, it is unknown whether Fc domain-modified aptamers have a longer elimination half-life than albumin-modified ones. Aptamer medicines are often exclusively provided through injection. However, because of the high proportion of the macromolecular moiety in the macromolecule-aptamer combination, increasing the subcutaneous dose of the aptamer moiety within a constant subcutaneous administration volume is difficult, limiting its therapeutic potential. As a result, it is critical to overcome the constraint of the dose increase space coming from macromolecular modification techniques.

Another method for modifying aptamers is to use tiny compounds with low molecular weight. Albumin, as previously stated, contains extensive hydrophobic interface cages that may bind particular low molecular weight chemical agents to create molecular complexes. Specific low molecular weight chemical agents can be used to alter aptamers and generate conjugates that bind albumin, resulting in molecular complexes with an average mass greater than the renal filtration cut-off threshold, hence increasing their half-life. Noncovalent binding allows medication attachment to albumin in this technique. Evans Blue (EB), for example, has a strong affinity for albumin and has been demonstrated to have a long half-life *in vivo* [65]. EB has been found to bind to the hydrophobic region of albumin, leading to the formation of a drug/albumin complex with an extended half-life in circulation and improved physiological stability. Due to this property, EB derivatives have been commonly utilized to enhance the pharmacokinetic properties of peptides and proteins. Researchers have utilized EB to modify Sgc8, an aptamer that specifically targets the PTK7 receptor [66]. Following the conjugation with EB, the aptamer showed a significantly prolonged half-life, and its targeting efficacy was markedly improved when compared to the original unconjugated aptamer. This modification with EB holds great promise for enhancing the therapeutic potential of aptamers and optimizing their in vivo performance. Furthermore, because albumin binds and transports fatty acids, they are often employed for long-term modification. For example, Patients with type 2 diabetes frequently require insulin shots to keep their blood sugar levels steady. However, numerous injections may cause compliance issues, limiting total therapy efficacy. To reduce dose frequency, long-acting glucagon-like peptide-1 receptor agonists (GLP-1RAs) such as liraglutide modified with palmitic acid (half-life of three days) and semaglutide modified with an octadecandioic acid derivative (half-life of seven days) have been created [67]. Jin et al. modified floxuridine homomeric oligonucleotide (LFU20) with a lipid having two fatty acid derivative tails [68]. By utilizing this technique, LFU20 was able to interact with the hydrophobic cavity of albumin, resulting in the formation of an LFU20/albumin complex. This complex exhibited enhanced tumor accumulation, thanks to the improved permeability and retention effect, and was subsequently internalized into the lysosomes of cancer cells. This approach holds great promise for targeted drug delivery and improving the therapeutic efficacy of anticancer agents.

When compared to PEGylation, the fatty acid modification techniques discussed above greatly enhance the fraction of aptamers. Fatty acids, on the other hand, can bind to fatty acid-binding proteins (FABPs), which are found in a variety of tissues throughout the body. This binding may cause drug loss inside those tissues, reducing the quantity of medication in circulation.

3.3 Cholesterol

Cholesterol conjugation (**Figure 5c**) is an alternate method for improving the pharmacokinetic properties of aptamers. Because low density lipoprotein (LDL) has a strong affinity for cholesterol, cholesterol is an excellent option for alteration. As a result, a cholesteryl-oligonucleotide (cholODN) was created by chemically bonding cholesterol to an aptamer's 5′ end [69]. Then, in contrast to its unaltered counterpart, the cholODN-LDL complex displayed exceptional resistance to nuclease hydrolysis in serum, resulting in a tenfold extension of half-life.

An RNA aptamer was modified with 2′-F-pyrimidine and connected to cholesterol in one research, resulting in a chol-aptamer [70]. This chol-aptamer was capable of cellular absorption and successfully prevented the replication of Hepatitis C viral RNAs. Importantly, both in vitro and in vivo tests found no evidence of chol-aptamer toxicity. Furthermore, the gene expression profile remained essentially unaltered, notably for typically implicated immune-related genes. Notably, mice who were given the chol-aptamer in vivo showed no obvious problems. The chol-aptamer displayed a considerably longer half-life and a ninefold decrease in plasma clearance rate when compared to unmodified aptamers. The addition of cholesterol to the aptamer improved its hydrophobicity, allowing it to bind to plasma lipoproteins and reduce renal clearance. Preclinical research has shown that cholesterol-conjugated aptamers had a longer circulation half-life and better biodistribution patterns. However, like with PEGylation, cholesterol conjugation may have an effect on the binding affinity of aptamers to their target molecules. As a result, the conjugation location and cholesterol moiety should be optimized.

3.4 Dialkyl lipid (DAG)

Willis et al. developed a way to increase the activity of an aptamer targeting vascular endothelial growth factor (VEGF) by conjugating it with diacylglycerol (DAG)

(**Figure 5d**). The aptamer's DAG moiety was attached to a lipid tail and integrated into a liposome's lipid bilayer. This DAG-aptamer-liposome complex performed better. Notably, as compared to the unmodified aptamer, the complex displayed considerably longer plasma retention duration.

4. Conclusions

Aptamers encounter problems such as lower in vivo stability and fast renal excretion. To address these difficulties, researchers used chemical changes to boost aptamer resistance to nucleases and *in vivo* stability. Modification can be accomplished either during the SELEX procedure (selection process) by adding functional groups to random libraries or after the SELEX methodology has been completed using solid-phase chemical synthesis. The latter approach is especially effective for adding phosphorothioate units that are resistant to nuclease digestion and inhibit fast renal filtration. The limited half-life extension provided by PEG components may require frequent subcutaneous injections, reducing compliance. Developing aptamers with higher proportion of the active aptamer component and employing low molecular weight modification approaches can enhance therapeutic efficacy.

Acknowledgements

This study was supported by Guangdong Basic and Applied Basic Research Foundation (2020A1515110630).

Conflict of interest

The authors declare no conflict of interest.

Author details

Yuan Ma[1*], Yihao Zhang[2], Zefeng Chen[1], Yuan Tian[1] and Ge Zhang[1*]

1 School of Chinese Medicine, Law Sau Fai Institute for Advancing Translational Medicine in Bone and Joint Diseases, Hong Kong Baptist University, Hong Kong SAR, China

2 Faculty of Medicine, School of Chinese Medicine, The Chinese University of Hong Kong, Hong Kong SAR, China

*Address all correspondence to: mayuan@hkbu.edu.hk and zhangge@hkbu.edu.hk

References

[1] Chen C, Zhou S, Cai Y, Tang F. Nucleic acid aptamer application in diagnosis and therapy of colorectal cancer based on cell-SELEX technology. NPJ Precision Oncology. 2017;**1**:37. DOI: 10.1038/s41698-017-0041-y

[2] Darmostuk M, Rimpelova S, Gbelcova H, Ruml T. Current approaches in SELEX: An update to aptamer selection technology. Biotechnology Advances. 2015;**33**:1141-1161. DOI: 10.1016/j.biotechadv.2015.02.008

[3] Amaya-González S, de Los Santos Álvarez N, Miranda-Ordieres AJ, Lobo-Castañón MJ. Aptamer binding to celiac disease-triggering hydrophobic proteins: A sensitive gluten detection approach. Analytical Chemistry. 2014;**86**:2733-2739. DOI: 10.1021/ac404151n

[4] Wei L, Cohen A. Spotlight commentary: Medicines use during pregnancy and harmful effects on offspring. British Journal of Clinical Pharmacology. 2019;**85**:1393. DOI: 10.1111/bcp.13931

[5] Ruckman J, Green LS, Beeson J, Waugh S, Gillette WL, Henninger DD, et al. 2'-Fluoropyrimidine RNA-based aptamers to the 165-amino acid form of vascular endothelial growth factor (VEGF165). Inhibition of receptor binding and VEGF-induced vascular permeability through interactions requiring the exon 7-encoded domain. The Journal of Biological Chemistry. 1998;**273**:20556-20567. DOI: 10.1074/jbc.273.32.20556

[6] Röthlisberger P, Hollenstein M. Aptamer chemistry. Advanced Drug Delivery Reviews. 2018;**134**:3-21. DOI: 10.1016/j.addr.2018.04.007

[7] Cheung YW, Röthlisberger P, Mechaly AE, Weber P, Levi-Acobas F, Lo Y, et al. Evolution of abiotic cubane chemistries in a nucleic acid aptamer allows selective recognition of a malaria biomarker. Proceedings of the National Academy of Sciences of the United States of America. 2020;**117**:16790-16798. DOI: 10.1073/pnas.2003267117

[8] Bayat P, Nosrati R, Alibolandi M, Rafatpanah H, Abnous K, Khedri M, et al. SELEX methods on the road to protein targeting with nucleic acid aptamers. Biochimie. 2018;**154**:132-155. DOI: 10.1016/j.biochi.2018.09.001

[9] Zhou J, Rossi J. Aptamers as targeted therapeutics: Current potential and challenges. Nature Reviews. Drug Discovery. 2017;**16**:181-202. DOI: 10.1038/nrd.2016.199

[10] Lee Y, Urban JH, Xu L, Sullenger BA, Lee J. 2'Fluoro modification differentially modulates the ability of RNAs to activate pattern recognition receptors. Nucleic Acid Therapeutics. 2016;**26**:173-182. DOI: 10.1089/nat.2015.0575

[11] Aaldering LJ, Tayeb H, Krishnan S, Fletcher S, Wilton SD, Veedu RN. Smart functional nucleic acid chimeras: Enabling tissue specific RNA targeting therapy. RNA Biology. 2015;**12**:412-425. DOI: 10.1080/15476286.2015.1017234

[12] Meek KN, Rangel AE, Heemstra JM. Enhancing aptamer function and stability via in vitro selection using modified nucleic acids. Methods. 2016;**106**:29-36. DOI: 10.1016/j.ymeth.2016.03.008

[13] Khvorova A, Watts JK. The chemical evolution of oligonucleotide therapies of clinical utility. Nature Biotechnology. 2017;**35**:238-248. DOI: 10.1038/nbt.3765

[14] Adler A, Forster N, Homann M, Göringer HU. Post-SELEX chemical optimization of a trypanosome-specific RNA aptamer. Combinatorial Chemistry & High Throughput Screening. 2008;**11**:16-23. DOI: 10.2174/138620708783398331

[15] Kratschmer C, Levy M. Effect of chemical modifications on Aptamer stability in serum. Nucleic Acid Therapeutics. 2017;**27**:335-344. DOI: 10.1089/nat.2017.0680

[16] Aurup H, Tuschl T, Benseler F, Ludwig J, Eckstein F. Oligonucleotide duplexes containing 2′-amino-2′-deoxycytidines: Thermal stability and chemical reactivity. Nucleic Acids Research. 1994;**22**:20-24. DOI: 10.1093/nar/22.1.20

[17] Kostyuk DA, Dragan SM, Lyakhov DL, Rechinsky VO, Tunitskaya VL, Chernov BK, et al. Mutants of T7 RNA polymerase that are able to synthesize both RNA and DNA. FEBS Letters. 1995;**369**:165-168. DOI: 10.1016/0014-5793(95)00732-o

[18] Sousa R, Padilla R. A mutant T7 RNA polymerase as a DNA polymerase. The EMBO Journal. 1995;**14**:4609-4621. DOI: 10.1002/j.1460-2075.1995.tb00140.x

[19] Huang Y, Eckstein F, Padilla R, Sousa R. Mechanism of ribose 2′-group discrimination by an RNA polymerase. Biochemistry. 1997;**36**:8231-8242. DOI: 10.1021/bi962674l

[20] Cummins LL, Owens SR, Risen LM, Lesnik EA, Freier SM, McGee D, et al. Characterization of fully 2′-modified oligoribonucleotide hetero- and homoduplex hybridization and nuclease sensitivity. Nucleic Acids Research. 1995;**23**:2019-2024. DOI: 10.1093/nar/23.11.2019

[21] Peng CG, Damha MJ. G-quadruplex induced stabilization by 2′-deoxy-2′-fluoro-D-arabinonucleic acids (2'F-ANA). Nucleic Acids Research. 2007;**35**:4977-4988. DOI: 10.1093/nar/gkm520

[22] Lin Y, Qiu Q, Gill SC, Jayasena SD. Modified RNA sequence pools for in vitro selection. Nucleic Acids Research. 1994;**22**:5229-5234. DOI: 10.1093/nar/22.24.5229

[23] Jellinek D, Green LS, Bell C, Lynott CK, Gill N, Vargeese C, et al. Potent 2′-amino-2′-deoxypyrimidine RNA inhibitors of basic fibroblast growth factor. Biochemistry. 1995;**34**:11363-11372. DOI: 10.1021/bi00036a009

[24] Green LS, Jellinek D, Bell C, Beebe LA, Feistner BD, Gill SC, et al. Nuclease-resistant nucleic acid ligands to vascular permeability factor/vascular endothelial growth factor. Chemistry & Biology. 1995;**2**:683-695. DOI: 10.1016/1074-5521(95)90032-2

[25] Frederiksen JK, Piccirilli JA. Separation of RNA phosphorothioate oligonucleotides by HPLC. Methods in Enzymology. 2009;**468**:289-309. DOI: 10.1016/s0076-6879(09)68014-9

[26] Hara RI, Yoshino R, Nukaga Y, Maeda Y, Sato K, Wada T. Synthesis and properties of DNA oligomers containing stereopure phosphorothioate linkages and C-5 modified deoxyuridine derivatives. RSC Advances. 2020;**10**:34006-34013. DOI: 10.1039/d0ra06970a

[27] Wu X, Zi Z, Bai H, Fu T, Yang C, Hu X, et al. DNA aptamer selected against pancreatic ductal adenocarcinoma for in vivo imaging and clinical tissue recognition. Theranostics. 2015;**5**:985-994. DOI: 10.7150/thno.11938

[28] Bardeesy N, DePinho RA. Pancreatic cancer biology and genetics. Nature Reviews. Cancer. 2002;**2**:897-909. DOI: 10.1038/nrc949

[29] Chen K, Liu J, Tong G, Liu B, Wang G, Liu H. Adipo8, a high-affinity DNA aptamer, can differentiate among adipocytes and inhibit intracellular lipid accumulation in vitro. Science China Chemistry. 2015;**58**:1612-1620. DOI: 10.1007/s11426-015-5367-0

[30] Volk DE, Lokesh GLR. Development of Phosphorothioate DNA and DNA Thioaptamers. Biomedicine. 2017;**5**:41. DOI: 10.3390/biomedicines5030041

[31] Chen Z, Luo H, Gubu A, Yu S, Zhang H, Dai H, et al. Chemically modified aptamers for improving binding affinity to the target proteins via enhanced non-covalent bonding. Frontiers in Cell and Development Biology. 2023;**11**:1091809. DOI: 10.3389/fcell.2023.1091809

[32] Jin B, Guo Z, Chen Z, Chen H, Li S, Deng Y, et al. Aptamers in cancer therapy: Problems and new breakthroughs. Journal of Materials Chemistry B. 2023;**11**:1609-1627. DOI: 10.1039/d2tb02579e

[33] Vater A, Klussmann S. Turning mirror-image oligonucleotides into drugs: The evolution of Spiegelmer(®) therapeutics. Drug Discovery Today. 2015;**20**:147-155. DOI: 10.1016/j.drudis.2014.09.004

[34] Wang Z, Xu W, Liu L, Zhu TF. A synthetic molecular system capable of mirror-image genetic replication and transcription. Nature Chemistry. 2016;**8**:698-704. DOI: 10.1038/nchem.2517

[35] Roccaro AM, Sacco A, Purschke WG, Moschetta M, Buchner K, Maasch C, et al. SDF-1 inhibition targets the bone marrow niche for cancer therapy. Cell Reports. 2014;**9**:118-128. DOI: 10.1016/j.celrep.2014.08.042

[36] Virgilio A, Varra M, Scuotto M, Capuozzo A, Irace C, Mayol L, et al. Expanding the potential of G-quadruplex structures: Formation of a heterochiral TBA analogue. Chembiochem. 2014;**15**:652-655. DOI: 10.1002/cbic.201300775

[37] Li K, Deng J, Jin H, Yang X, Fan X, Li L, et al. Chemical modification improves the stability of the DNA aptamer GBI-10 and its affinity towards tenascin-C. Organic & Biomolecular Chemistry. 2017;**15**:1174-1182. DOI: 10.1039/c6ob02577c

[38] Li L, Hou J, Liu X, Guo Y, Wu Y, Zhang L, et al. Nucleolin-targeting liposomes guided by aptamer AS1411 for the delivery of siRNA for the treatment of malignant melanomas. Biomaterials. 2014;**35**:3840-3850. DOI: 10.1016/j.biomaterials.2014.01.019

[39] Lee JH, Canny MD, De Erkenez A, Krilleke D, Ng YS, Shima DT, et al. A therapeutic aptamer inhibits angiogenesis by specifically targeting the heparin binding domain of VEGF165. Proceedings of the National Academy of Sciences of the United States of America. 2005;**102**:18902-18907. DOI: 10.1073/pnas.0509069102

[40] Rusconi CP, Scardino E, Layzer J, Pitoc GA, Ortel TL, Monroe D, et al. RNA aptamers as reversible antagonists of coagulation factor IXa. Nature. 2002;**419**:90-94. DOI: 10.1038/nature00963

[41] Di Giusto DA, King GC. Construction, stability, and activity of multivalent circular anticoagulant aptamers. The Journal of Biological

Chemistry. 2004;**279**:46483-46489. DOI: 10.1074/jbc.M408037200

[42] Tan J, Yang N, Hu Z, Su J, Zhong J, Yang Y, et al. Aptamer-functionalized fluorescent silica nanoparticles for highly sensitive detection of leukemia cells. Nanoscale Research Letters. 2016;**11**:298. DOI: 10.1186/s11671-016-1512-8

[43] Zhang XJ, Zhao Z, Wang X, Su MH, Ai L, Li Y, et al. A versatile strategy for convenient circular bivalent functional nucleic acids construction. National Science Review. 2023;**10**:nwac107. DOI: 10.1093/nsr/nwac107

[44] Zhou F, Wang P, Peng Y, Zhang P, Huang Q, Sun W, et al. Molecular engineering-based Aptamer-drug conjugates with accurate Tunability of drug ratios for drug combination targeted cancer therapy. Angewandte Chemie (International Ed. in English). 2019;**58**:11661-11665. DOI: 10.1002/anie.201903807

[45] Vaganov AA, Taranushenko TE, LuzanNA, ShchugorevaIA, KolovskayaOS, Artyushenko PV, et al. Aptamers regulating the hemostasis system. Molecules. 2022;**27**:8593. DOI: 10.3390/molecules27238593

[46] Park EJ, Sun Kim M, Suk Lee H, Choon Lee K, Hee ND. Differences in electrophoretic behavior between linear and branched PEG-conjugated proteins. Electrophoresis. 2015;**36**:918-923. DOI: 10.1002/elps.201400539

[47] Zhang Y, Zhang H, Chan DWH, Ma Y, Lu A, Yu S, et al. Strategies for developing long-lasting therapeutic nucleic acid aptamer targeting circulating protein: The present and the future. Frontiers in Cell and Development Biology. 2022;**10**:1048148. DOI: 10.3389/fcell.2022.1048148

[48] Kaminskas LM, Kelly BD, McLeod VM, Boyd BJ, Krippner GY, Williams ED, et al. Pharmacokinetics and tumor disposition of PEGylated, methotrexate conjugated poly-l-lysine dendrimers. Molecular Pharmaceutics. 2009;**6**:1190-1204. DOI: 10.1021/mp900049a

[49] Suk JS, Xu Q, Kim N, Hanes J, Ensign LM. PEGylation as a strategy for improving nanoparticle-based drug and gene delivery. Advanced Drug Delivery Reviews. 2016;**99**:28-51. DOI: 10.1016/j.addr.2015.09.012

[50] Gilbert JC, DeFeo-Fraulini T, Hutabarat RM, Horvath CJ, Merlino PG, MarshHN, etal. First-in-humanevaluation of anti von Willebrand factor therapeutic aptamer ARC1779 in healthy volunteers. Circulation. 2007;**116**:2678-2686. DOI: 10.1161/circulationaha.107.724864

[51] Siller-Matula JM, Merhi Y, Tanguay JF, Duerschmied D, Wagner DD, McGinness KE, et al. ARC15105 is a potent antagonist of von Willebrand factor mediated platelet activation and adhesion. Arteriosclerosis, Thrombosis, and Vascular Biology. 2012;**32**:902-909. DOI: 10.1161/atvbaha.111.237529

[52] Altiok EI, Browne S, Khuc E, Moran EP, Qiu F, Zhou K, et al. sFlt multivalent conjugates inhibit angiogenesis and improve half-life In vivo. PLoS One. 2016;**11**:e0155990. DOI: 10.1371/journal.pone.0155990

[53] Steurer M, Montillo M, Scarfò L, Mauro FR, Andel J, Wildner S, et al. Olaptesed pegol (NOX-A12) with bendamustine and rituximab: A phase IIa study in patients with relapsed/refractory chronic lymphocytic leukemia. Haematologica. 2019;**104**:2053-2060. DOI: 10.3324/haematol.2018.205930

[54] Boyce M, Warrington S, Cortezi B, Zöllner S, Vauléon S, Swinkels DW,

et al. Safety, pharmacokinetics and pharmacodynamics of the anti-hepcidin Spiegelmer lexaptepid pegol in healthy subjects. British Journal of Pharmacology. 2016;**173**:1580-1588. DOI: 10.1111/bph.13433

[55] Yin S, Wang Y, Zhang B, Qu Y, Liu Y, Dai S, et al. Engineered human heavy-chain ferritin with half-life extension and tumor targeting by PAS and RGDK peptide functionalization. Pharmaceutics. 2021;**13**:521. DOI: 10.3390/pharmaceutics13040521

[56] Zhu S, Xing H, Gordiichuk P, Park J, Mirkin CA. PLGA spherical nucleic acids. Advanced Materials. 2018;**30**:e1707113. DOI: 10.1002/adma.201707113

[57] van Witteloostuijn SB, Pedersen SL, Jensen KJ. Half-life extension of biopharmaceuticals using chemical methods: Alternatives to PEGylation. ChemMedChem. 2016;**11**:2474-2495. DOI: 10.1002/cmdc.201600374

[58] Ibrahim M, Ramadan E, Elsadek NE, Emam SE, Shimizu T, Ando H, et al. Polyethylene glycol (PEG): The nature, immunogenicity, and role in the hypersensitivity of PEGylated products. Journal of Controlled Release. 2022;**351**:215-230. DOI: 10.1016/j.jconrel.2022.09.031

[59] Vincent JL, Russell JA, Jacob M, Martin G, Guidet B, Wernerman J, et al. Albumin administration in the acutely ill: What is new and where next? Critical Care. 2014;**18**:231. DOI: 10.1186/cc13991

[60] Spada A, Emami J, Tuszynski JA, Lavasanifar A. The uniqueness of albumin as a carrier in Nanodrug delivery. Molecular Pharmaceutics. 2021;**18**:1862-1894. DOI: 10.1021/acs.molpharmaceut.1c00046

[61] Sleep D. Albumin and its application in drug delivery. Expert Opinion on Drug Delivery. 2015;**12**:793-812. DOI: 10.1517/17425247.2015.993313

[62] Kuhlmann M, Hamming JBR, Voldum A, Tsakiridou G, Larsen MT, Schmøkel JS, et al. An albumin-oligonucleotide assembly for potential combinatorial drug delivery and half-life extension applications. Molecular Therapy—Nucleic Acids. 2017;**9**:284-293. DOI: 10.1016/j.omtn.2017.10.004

[63] Schmøkel J, Voldum A, Tsakiridou G, Kuhlmann M, Cameron J, Sørensen ES, et al. Site-selective conjugation of an anticoagulant aptamer to recombinant albumins and maintenance of neonatal fc receptor binding. Nanotechnology. 2017;**28**:204004. DOI: 10.1088/1361-6528/aa6a9b

[64] Zong Y, Tan X, Xiao J, Zhang X, Xia X, Sun H. Half-life extension of porcine interferon-α by fusion to the IgG-binding domain of streptococcal G protein. Protein Expression and Purification. 2019;**153**:53-58. DOI: 10.1016/j.pep.2018.08.012

[65] Wen X, Xu P, Shi M, Liu J, Zeng X, Zhang Y, et al. Evans blue-modified radiolabeled fibroblast activation protein inhibitor as long-acting cancer therapeutics. Theranostics. 2022;**12**:422-433. DOI: 10.7150/thno.68182

[66] Ding D, Yang C, Lv C, Li J, Tan W. Improving tumor accumulation of Aptamers by prolonged blood circulation. Analytical Chemistry. 2020;**92**:4108-4114. DOI: 10.1021/acs.analchem.9b05878

[67] Nauck MA, Quast DR, Wefers J, Meier JJ. GLP-1 receptor agonists in the treatment of type 2 diabetes - state-of-the-art. Molecular Metabolism. 2021;**46**:101102. DOI: 10.1016/j.molmet.2020.101102

[68] Jin C, Zhang H, Zou J, Liu Y, Zhang L, Li F, et al. Floxuridine Homomeric oligonucleotides "hitchhike" with albumin In situ for cancer chemotherapy. Angewandte Chemie (International Ed. in English). 2018;**57**:8994-8997. DOI: 10.1002/anie.201804156

[69] de Smidt PC, Le Doan T, de Falco S, van Berkel TJ. Association of antisense oligonucleotides with lipoproteins prolongs the plasma half-life and modifies the tissue distribution. Nucleic Acids Research. 1991;**19**:4695-4700. DOI: 10.1093/nar/19.17.4695

[70] Lee CH, Lee SH, Kim JH, Noh YH, Noh GJ, Lee SW. Pharmacokinetics of a cholesterol-conjugated Aptamer against the hepatitis C virus (HCV) NS5B protein. Molecular Therapy—Nucleic Acids. 2015;**4**:e254. DOI: 10.1038/mtna.2015.30

Chapter 7

Bioactive Indanes: Development and Validation of a Bioanalytical Method of LC-MS/MS for the Determination of PH46A, a New Potential Anti-Inflammatory Agent, in Human Plasma, Urine and Faeces

Tao Zhang, Gaia A. Scalabrino, Neil Frankish and Helen Sheridan

Abstract

PH46A, a new chemical entity developed by our group, has shown potent anti-inflammatory activities through various pre-preclinical studies. The aim of this work was to develop and validate a sensitive and robust LC-MS/MS analytical method to determine the levels of PH46 in human plasma, urine and faeces. The linearity (0.5–500 ng/mL for plasma/urine, and 10–2000 ng/g for human faeces), accuracy (within $100 \pm 15\%$ for plasma/urine or $100 \pm 20\%$ for faeces), precision ($\leq 15\%$ CV for plasma/urine or $\leq 20\%$ CV for faeces) and the method's specificity were demonstrated to be acceptable. No significant matrix effects or carry-over was observed for PH46 and IStd, and the recovery was consistent. About 10- and 100-fold dilutions in control matrix were found not to affect the assays' performance. PH46 was proven to be stable: at room temperature for >24 hrs in plasma through 3 freeze-thaw cycles, at –20°C for 83 days in plasma/32 days in urine/33 days in faeces, and at –80°C for 154 days in plasma/33 days in faeces. The re-injection reproducibility of PH46 in matrix extracts was at least 239 hrs at 4°C in plasma/25 days in urine/6.5 days in faeces. This method was successfully applied to the pharmacokinetic evaluation of the Phase I clinical studies.

Keywords: bioanalytical, development, validation, LC-MS/MS, PH46A, human plasma, urine, faeces

1. Introduction

The therapeutic effect of indane derived molecules has been clinically evident for treatment of many disease conditions, ranging from inflammation [1], cancer [2], neurological conditions [3] to HIV [4]. Several classes of indane dimers have been developed, characterised and investigated by our research group [5–7] for various biological activities, including smooth muscle relaxation, mediator release inhibition and inflammatory conditions [8–14]. In particular, A lead, first-in-class molecule, [6-(Methylamino)hexane-1,2,3,4,5-pentanol 4-(((1S,2S)-1-hydroxy-2,3-dihydro-1H,1′H-[2,2-biinden]-2-yl)methyl)benzoate (PH46A) (**Figure 1**) with S, S configuration [15] has been considered as a potential new treatment for inflammatory bowel disease (IBD) based on the observation of its biological effect in two different well-established preclinical models of murine colitis: the acute dextran sodium sulphate model and the chronic and spontaneous Interleukin-10 (IL-$10^{-/-}$) knock-out mouse model. During the course of our work, PH46A was subject to a range of preclinical studies [16–19] prior to entering a Phase I clinical trial which has recently been completed [20].

This manuscript describes the development and validation of a sensitive and specific liquid chromatography-tandem mass spectrometry (LC-MS/MS) bioanalytical method for determining PH46 (the free acid form of PH46A salt) (**Figure 1**) in human plasma, urine and faeces samples according to the US Food and Drug Administration (FDA) Guidance Document on Bioanalytical Method Validation [21] and the European Medicines Agency (EMA) Guidelines on Bioanalytical Method validation [22]. The method was subsequently used to analyse the clinical samples from healthy volunteers in the Phase 1 trial [20]. The lower limit of quantification (LLOQ) in plasma and urine was 0.5 ng/mL and the LLOQ in faeces was 10 ng/g faecal equivalent.

2. Results and discussion

2.1 Stability of PH46 and IStd in stored stock solutions

The mean accuracy of the stored solutions compared to freshly prepared solutions met the acceptance criteria. Both PH46 and Compound 1 (Internal Standard, IStd) (**Figure 1**) stock solutions were found to be stable at 4°C for at least 200 and 250 days, respectively. The stability of IStd working solutions for at least 192 days at 4°C, and PH46 stock solutions for at least 24 h at room temperature (RT) was demonstrated.

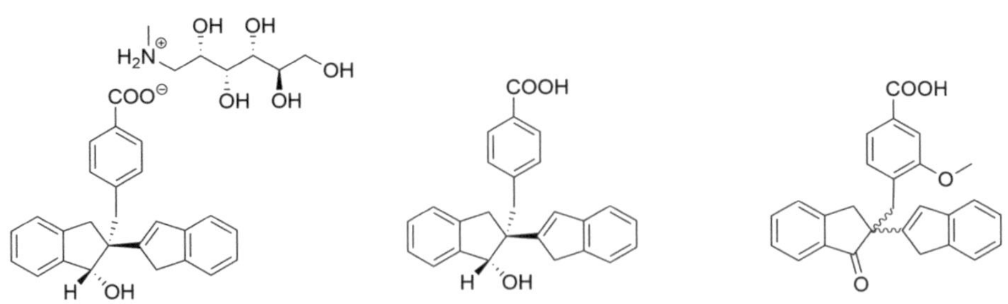

PH46A **PH46** **Compound 1 (IStd)**

Figure 1.
Chemical structures of PH46A, PH46 and compound 1 (internal standard, IStd).

2.2 Linearity and specificity

The calibration data from reported human plasma (12 batches), urine (3 batches) and faeces (3 batches) standards over a range of 0.5–500 ng/mL (plasma or urine) or 10–2000 ng/g (faecal equivalent), duplicate run at each concertation, were analysed. The data are presented in **Table 1** for human plasma and **Table 2** for human urine and faeces batches.

In all cases, all concentrations determined for these standards met the acceptance criteria being at least 75% of standards [including at least one replicate at the LLOQ and the upper limit of quantification (ULOQ) levels] used to construct each calibration line met the acceptance criterion of the determined concentrations being within 100 ± 15% (plasma and urine batches) or 100 ± 20% (faeces batches) of the nominal concentrations (100 ± 20% for plasma and urine batches or 100 ± 25% for faeces batches of the nominal concentration at the LLOQ).

Regression analysis of the peak area ratios of PH46:IStd against the concentration showed good linearity for human plasma, urine and faeces over the range of concentration tested (0.5–500 ng/mL for plasma/urine samples and 10–2000 ng/g faecal equivalent for faeces samples) using a linear regression with a weighting factor of $1/x^2$ (**Tables 3** and **4**). All calculated concentrations for these standards met the acceptance criteria.

The quality control (QC) sample data for the supporting QC samples are presented in **Table 5**, which met the acceptance criteria. The selectivity of the assay for PH46 and IStd was determined by extraction and analysis of the following samples: one double blank (DB) sample (control matrix only without PH46 or IStd) from six independent sources of control matrix; three single blank (SB) samples (control matrix with IStd only) in a single source of control matrix; three ULOQ samples (no IStd) in the same source of control matrix as for the SB samples. The assay specificity demonstrated there were no significant interfering substances (IStd, PH46 or any impurity) at the retention times of PH46 and IStd, respectively. Samples containing either PH46 or IStd showed no significant interfering substances at the retention time of the other compound. Therefore, the assays were deemed to be specific to PH46. Representative chromatograms of human plasma extracts containing PH46 and IStd (LLOQ and ULOQ) are shown in **Figure 2**.

2.3 Assay recovery and matrix effects

For PH46 and IStd in plasma, the recovery was consistent. When the concentration of PH46 at 1.25 ng/mL, the IStd-normalised Matric Factors (MFs) (six sources) were calculated: 1.40, 1.35, 1.46, 1.51, 1.57, 1.25, 1.37 and the associated precision was determined to be 7.8%. When the PH46 concentration at 400 ng/mL, the IStd-normalised MFs were 1.35, 1.26, 1.45, 1.38, 1.44, 1.21, 1.25 and the corresponding precision was found to be 7.2%. These results confirmed that the matrix effects met the acceptance criteria, and no significant matrix effect was present for PH46 and IStd in human plasma by the current method.

2.4 Assay carry-over and matrix dilution

For human plasma, urine and faeces samples, no significant carry-over was observed in the matrix blank and solvent samples injected after a ULOQ sample for PH46 or IStd using needle-wash solution: [H_2O:acetonitrile (ACN):trifluoroacetic acid

Batch	Nominal concentration of PH46 (ng/mL)								Calibration curve parameters		
	0.500	**1.00**	**3.25**	**12.5**	**50.0**	**150**	**450**	**500**	**Slope**	**Intercept**	**R^2**
1	0.524 0.458	1.08 1.01	2.99 3.34	13.5 11.3	51.8 50.1	158 157	444 414	469 513	0.05576	0.002248	0.9951
2	0.489 0.534	0.894 1.03	2.99 3.31	15.6* 14.7*	55.0 52.2	185* 171	400 441	471 NR	0.07431	0.005518	0.9908
4	0.493 0.510	0.929 1.03	3.28 3.41	13.3 12.8	53.7 52.0	159 145	445 404	468 458	0.09615	0.002045	0.9958
5	0.454 0.548	0.897 1.04	3.63 3.46	12.2 12.2	48.5 49.6	157 156	444 442	466 484	0.08515	0.007061	0.9948
6	0.563 0.427	1.07 0.964	3.28 3.22	13.7 12.7	51.6 46.7	166 147	420 372*	445 397*	0.1433	0.001421	0.9909
7	0.521 0.471	1.08 0.931	3.48 3.15	14.6* 13.9	53.3 48.3	163 152	427 386	457 401*	0.1846	0.006788	0.9919
8	0.425 0.577	0.935 1.03	3.18 3.57	12.3 13.6	50.4 53.7	145 163	408 443	460 465	0.1267	0.002473	0.9909
9	0.500 0.490	1.01 1.02	3.22 3.29	12.7 13.3	52.0 50.1	150 153	459 425	491 449	0.06133	0.001111	0.9981
10	0.495 0.496	0.986 1.03	3.28 3.42	12.5 12.6	50.7 52.4	148 153	426 446	468 492	0.05657	0.002131	0.9987
11	0.465 0.540	0.959 0.964	3.52 3.56	12.6 12.7	49.1 54.4	147 145	406 465	486 471	0.04653	0.003935	0.9952
12	0.505 0.485	1.03 0.982	3.48 3.17	13.3 13.4	51.3 49.9	155 148	419 416	478 486	0.07467	0.005944	0.9971
Mean	0.499	0.996	3.33	12.9	51.2	154	428	472	0.09137	0.003698	0.9945
Precision (%)	8.0	5.6	5.3	5.0	4.1	4.8	4.8	3.5	–	—	—
Accuracy (%)	99.8	99.6	102.5	103.2	102.4	102.7	95.1	94.4	—	—	—

–: not applicable.
**Outside acceptance criteria (100 ± 15%), value not used in statistical calculations or regression analysis. NR: no result as no internal standard peak detected in sample, value not used in statistical calculations.*

Table 1.
Calibration curve data and parameters for PH46 in human plasma.

(TFA) (25:75:0.1, *v/v/v*); H_2O:ACN:formic acid (FA):TFA (90:10:0.1:0.005, *v/v/v/v*)]. The accuracy and precision for plasma and urine samples prepared at 4000 ng/mL or faeces samples at 16000 ng/g eq., and diluted at 10- and 100-fold, also met the acceptance criteria (**Table 6**). The results showed that dilutions of samples in control plasma, urine and homogenised faeces had no effect on the accuracy and precision of the method.

2.5 Intra- and inter-batch assay accuracy and precision

The intra-batch accuracy and precision of the assay for PH46 in plasma, urine and faeces met the acceptance criteria at each of the four concentrations assessed. The inter-batch accuracy and precision for PH46 in plasma also meet the acceptance criteria on each occasion (**Table 7**).

Urine	Batch	Nominal concentration of PH46 (ng/mL)								Calibration curve parameters		
		0.500	**1.00**	**3.25**	**12.5**	**50.0**	**150**	**450**	**500**	**Slope**	**Intercept**	**R^2**
	1	0.525 0.502	1.02 0.923	2.60* 2.90	10.7 11.0	49.7 48.6	153 153	471 513	538 554	0.03028	−0.002197	0.9910
	4	0.503 0.313*	1.07 0.983	2.80 2.69*	10.8 11.1	48.2 50.4	152 156	482 477	536 556	0.03211	−0.001705	0.9920
	5	0.471 0.557	0.948 0.898	2.61* 3.58	14.0 12.8	50.7 53.5	161 156	423 417	435 460	0.03061	0.0004537	0.9909
	Mean	0.512	0.974	3.09	11.7	50.2	155	464	513	0.03100	−0.001149	0.9913
	Precision (%)	6.2	6.6	13.7	11.5	3.8	2.1	8.0	10.2	—	—	—
	Accuracy (%)	102.4	97.4	95.1	93.6	100.4	103.3	103.1	102.6	—	—	—
Faeces	**Batch**	**Nominal concentration of PH46 (ng/g eq.)**								**Calibration curve parameters**		
		10.0	**20.0**	**48.0**	**120**	**280**	**720**	**1800**	**2000**	**Slope**	**Intercept**	**R^2**
	2	9.54 10.4	18.5 21.9	43.9 49.1	115 139	254 267	708 793	1930 1810	1890 1930	0.01759	0.01151	0.9922
	3	10.2 9.15	19.1 23.8	45.0 49.1	112 124	251 287	693 696	2090 1840	1900 2000	0.01539	0.01445	0.9908
	6	10.1 9.73	20.6 10.2*	42.9 51.3	74.4* 127	276 315	693 441*	1750 1920	1850 1860	0.01116	−0.002342	0.9939
	Mean	9.85	20.8	46.9	123	275	717	1890	1910	0.01471	0.007873	0.9923
	Precision (%)	4.7	10.3	7.2	8.7	8.7	6.0	6.3	2.9	—	—	—
	Accuracy (%)	98.5	104.1	97.7	102.5	98.2	99.6	105.1	95.5	—	—	—

–: not applicable.
**Outside acceptance criteria 100 ± 15% (urine) or 100 ± 20% (faeces) [100 ± 20% (urine) or 100 ± 25% (faeces) at the LLOQ], value not used in regression analysis. LLOQ: at the lower limit of quantification.*

Table 2.
Calibration curve data and parameters for PH46 in human urine and faeces.

Nominal conc. of PH46 (ng/mL)	Occasion 1			Occasion 2			Occasion 3		
	Response	Calculated conc. (ng/mL)	Bias (%)	Response	Calculated conc. (ng/mL)	Bias (%)	Response	Calculated conc. (ng/mL)	Bias (%)
0.500	0.031488	0.524	4.8	0.041840	0.489	−2.2	0.045759	0.454	−9.2
	0.027788	0.458	−8.4	0.045210	0.534	6.8	0.053705	0.548	9.6
1.00	0.062580	1.08	8.0	0.071948	0.894	−10.6	0.083474	0.897	−10.3
	0.058307	1.01	1.0	0.082009	1.03	3.0	0.095815	1.04	4.0
3.25	0.168746	2.99	−8.0	0.227887	2.99	−8.0	0.316055	3.63	11.7
	0.188249	3.34	2.8	0.251369	3.31	1.8	0.301471	3.46	6.5
12.5	0.756801	13.5	8.0	1.166293	15.6*	24.8*	1.049172	12.2	−2.4
	0.633890	11.3	−9.6	1.101343	14.7*	17.6*	1.043108	12.2	−2.4
50.0	2.888743	51.8	3.6	4.093857	55.0	10.0	4.138322	48.5	−3.0
	2.798080	50.1	0.2	3.883057	52.2	4.4	4.230480	49.6	−0.8
150	8.833344	158	5.3	13.718101	185*	23.3*	13.394936	157	4.7
	8.769691	157	4.7	12.682625	171	14.0	13.315633	156	4.0
450	24.759200	444	−1.3	29.696339	400	−11.1	37.845875	444	−1.3
	23.116439	414	−8.0	32.792890	441	−2.0	37.649477	442	−1.8
500	26.174887	469	−6.2	34.993741	471	−5.8	39.725235	466	−6.8
	28.612686	513	2.6	—	—	—	41.206685	484	−3.2
Slope	0.05576			0.07431			0.08515		
Intercept	0.002248			0.005518			0.007061		
R^2	0.9951			0.9908			0.9948		

–: no result, no internal standard detected in sample. R^2: coefficient of determination. Bias: difference between determined concentration and nominal concentration. Conc.: concentration.
**Value outside acceptance criteria (100 ± 15%) and not used in regression analysis.*

Table 3.
Assay linearity for PH46 in human plasma.

Nominal conc. (ng/mL)	PH46 in human urine			PH46 in human faeces			
	Response	Calculated conc. (ng/mL)	Bias (%)	Nominal conc. (ng/g eq.)	Response	Calculated conc. (ng/g eq.)	Bias (%)
0.500	0.013704	0.525	5.0	10.0	0.179251	9.54	−4.6
	0.012990	0.502	0.4		0.195100	10.4	4.0
1.00	0.028823	1.02	2.0	20.0	0.336200	18.5	−7.5
	0.025742	0.923	−7.7		0.397292	21.9	9.5
3.25	0.076650	2.60*	−20.0*	48.0	0.784065	43.9	−8.5
	0.085737	2.90	−10.8		0.874742	49.1	2.3
12.5	0.320860	10.7	−14.4	120	2.033762	115	−4.2
	0.329679	11.0	−12.0		2.459854	139	15.8
50.0	0.502113	49.7	−0.6	280	4.485738	254	−9.3
	1.470794	48.6	−2.8		4.704624	267	−4.6
150	4.622468	153	2.0	720	12.464152	708	−1.7
	4.632629	153	2.0		13.952398	793	10.1
450	14.258525	471	4.7	1800	33.899934	1930	7.2
	15.531203	513	14.0		31.771859	1810	0.6
500	16.297231	538	7.6	2000	33.258315	1890	−5.5
	16.758430	554	10.8		33.933302	1930	−3.5
Slope	0.03028				0.01759		
Intercept	−0.002197				0.01151		
R^2	0.9910				0.9922		

Bias: difference between determined concentration and nominal concentration. Conc.: concentration.
**Value outside acceptance criteria 100 ± 15% (urine) and not used in regression analysis.*

Table 4.
Assay linearity for PH46 in human urine and faeces.

2.6 Stability experiments of PH46 in matrix

The results of different stability experiments are summarised in **Table 8** with the detailed data presented in **Tables 9–11**.

The mean stability results of PH46 in human plasma, at low, high and diluted concentrations, after at least one-month (33 days) storage at −20°C did not meet the acceptance criteria. This experiment was repeated after 35 days storage and similar results were obtained (**Table 11**). The data were unexpected as no stability issues had been observed in the previous studies of PH46 in dog and rat plasma [16]. Stability studies of PH46 in human plasma at −80°C, was subsequently assessed after at least one month (30 days) storage alongside the assessment of the −20°C stability after at least two months (83 days) storage (**Table 11**). The mean stability results at all concentration levels met the acceptance criteria for both storage temperatures and durations. The data generated for the two-month stability timepoint at −20°C contradict that of the one-month timepoint, but provide confidence that there should not be stability issue at −20°C. At one-month timepoint at −20°C, fresh calibration

Nominal conc. (ng/mL)		1.25	15	400
PH46 in plasma	Batch 6	1.22	15.3	354
		1.20	14.9	368
	Batch 7	1.20	15.4	341
		1.17	14.6	347
	Batch 8	1.14	14.7	387
		1.35	14.5	382
	Batch 9	1.16	15.6	392
		1.28	15.6	378
	Batch 10	1.28	15.0	400
		1.22	15.5	388
	Batch 11	1.33	16.1	362
		1.18	15.0	410
	Batch 12	1.24	14.8	373
		1.30	15.3	374
	Mean	1.23	15.2	375
	Precision (%)	5.3	3.0	5.3
	Accuracy (%)	98.4	101.3	93.8
Nominal conc. (ng/mL)		**1.25**	**15**	**400**
PH46 in urine	Batch 5	1.24	15.1	412
		1.28	9.23*	388
	Mean	1.26	12.2	400
	Precision (%)	—	—	—
	Accuracy (%)	100.8	81.3	100.0
Nominal conc. (ng/g eq.)		**25.0**	**100**	**1600**
PH46 in faeces	Batch 6	21.2	69.4*	1180*
		25.2	91.1	1780
	Mean	23.2	80.3	1480
	Precision (%)	—	—	—
	Accuracy (%)	92.8	80.3	92.5

-: no applicable. Conc.: concentration.
**Outside acceptance criteria value included in statistical analysis.*

Table 5.
Quality control data relating to PH46 in human plasma, urine and faeces.

standard (CS) and QC stock solutions were prepared and tested to ensure the stocks were suitable for use. The stock solutions were then used to prepare fresh bulk CSs and QC samples in control matrix., and the stability samples were extracted alongside these fresh CS and QC samples. The acceptance criteria for both CSs and supporting QC samples were met for each of the stability batches, therefore giving no reason to suspect the failing stability data after one-month storage at −20°C.

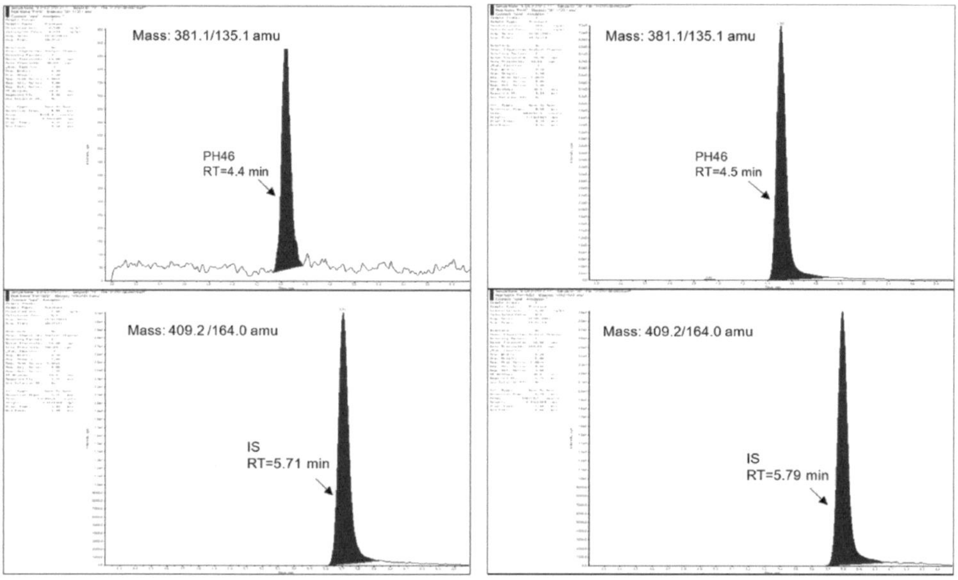

Figure 2.
Chromatograms of a human plasma extract (left) containing PH46 (LLOQ, 0.5 ng/mL) & internal standard and a human plasma extract (right) containing PH46 (ULOQ, 500 ng/mL) & internal standard.

Replicate	Plasma		Urine		Faeces	
	DF		DF		DF	
	10	100	10	100	10	100
1	3550	4260	4520	3940	16,800	15,600
2	3950	3660	4530	3910	16,500	15,600
3	3160	3830	4480	4100	17,800	19,400
4	3450	5000	4430	4050	18,700	16,200
5	4210	3320	4360	4000	17,100	19,400
6	3890	4310	4540	3820	18,100	14,600
Mean	3700	4060	4480	3970	17,500	16,800
Precision (%)	10.4	14.6	1.6	2.5	4.8	12.4
Accuracy (%)	92.5	101.5	112.0	99.3	109.4	105.0

Initial concentration of PH46: 4000 ng/mL (plasma and urine) or 16,000 ng/g eq. (faeces). DF: dilution factor.

Table 6.
Effects of dilution of PH46 with human plasma, urine and faeces homogenate.

At the one-month timepoint for −80°C and two-month timepoint for −20°C, a further fresh set of CS and QC stock solutions were made and used to prepare the fresh bulk CS and QC samples extracted alongside the stability samples. The acceptance criteria for these CSs and supporting QC samples were met. As the stability samples stored at −20°C and −80°C extracted in this batch also met the acceptance criteria, this demonstrates that both sets of samples prepared at different times were appropriate for use. Although there is still no explanation for the anomalous results at

	Nominal conc. (ng/mL)	0.5			1.25			15			400		
	Occasion	1	2	3	1	2	3	1	2	3	1	2	3
A	Intra-assay Mean (n = 6)	0.443	0.487	0.476	1.21	1.30	1.22	15.7	14.0	14.8	404	354	371
	Intra-assay precision (%)	10.0	4.6	14.5	6.8	6.8	4.5	6.8	5.2	4.4	5.5	3.8	5.1
	Intra-assay accuracy (%)	88.6	97.4	95.2	96.8	104.0	97.6	104.7	93.3	98.7	101.0	88.5	92.8
	Inter-assay Mean		0.469			1.24			14.8		376		
	Inter-assay precision (%)		10.6			6.7			7.2		7.4		
	Inter-assay accuracy (%)		93.8			99.2			98.7		94.0		
B	**Nominal conc. (ng/mL)**		**0.5**			**1.25**			**15**		**400**		
	Intra-assay mean (n = 6)		0.566			1.38			16.7		429		
	Intra-assay precision (%)		6.4			4.1			1.9		1.5		
	Intra-assay accuracy (%)		113.2			110.4			111.3		107.3		
C	**Nominal conc. (ng/g eq.)**		**10**			**25**			**100**		**1600**		
	Intra-assay mean (n = 6)		9.56			26.5			111		1500		
	Intra-assay precision (%)		7.3			8.5			11.0		5.7		
	Intra-assay accuracy (%)		95.6			106.0			111.0		93.8		

A: human plasma assay. B: human urine assay. C: human faeces assay. Conc.: concentration.

Table 7.
Intra- and inter-assay accuracy and precision for PH46 in human plasma, urine, and faeces.

one-month timepoint for −20°C storage, it does provide confidence that there is not a stability issue for PH46 in human plasma at −20°C for the timeframe tested (**Table 11**). After at least four months (153 days) storage at −20°C, the mean stability results met the acceptance criteria at high and diluted concentrations but did not meet at the low concentration. The low concentration samples were repeated and the failure to meet the acceptance criteria was confirmed. The mean stability results, after storing PH46 in human plasma −80°C for at least three months (100 days) and five months (154 days) met the acceptance criteria at all levels of low, high and diluted concentration (**Table 11**).

Following the successful method establishment, this validated bioanalytical method was applied to determine PH46 in human samples obtained from the healthy volunteering during the phase I clinical study (ISRCTN90725219) [20].

Stability study	Results
Short-term frozen storage stability and freeze/thaw stability of PH46 in matrix	At low, high and diluted concentrations, the mean stability results (after 3 freeze/thaw cycles in plasma, **Table 9A**, one month storage at −20°C and −80°C in urine and faeces, **Table 10A** and **B**) met the acceptance criteria.
Ambient room temperature stability of PH46	The results of the 24-h ambient room temperature stability of PH46 in human plasma at low, high and dilution concentrations also met the acceptance criteria (**Table 9B**).
Stability of PH46 in human plasma, urine and faeces extracts (re-injection reproducibility)	The mean reinjection reproducibility of PH46 extracts of plasma for 239 h, urine for 25 days and faeces for 6.5 days, stored in an autosampler at 4°C before being re-injected, also met the acceptance criteria (**Tables 9C** and **10C, D**).
Extended frozen storage stability	PH46 is stable in human plasma after two months (83 days) at −20 to 80°C and at least 5 months (154 days) at −80°C (**Table 11**).

Table 8.
Summary of stability results of PH46 in human plasma, urine and faeces.

	0.5*		1.25*		400*		4000*, #	
A.	B.L.	3 Cycles	B.L.	3 Cycles	B.L.	3 Cycles	B.L.	3 Cycles
Mean (n = 6)	–	–	1.30	1.22	354	365	3750	3510
Precision (%)	–	–	6.8	5.8	3.8	7.2	2.5	6.4
Accuracy (%)	–	–	97.6		91.3		87.8	
B.	**B.L.**	**24 h**	**B.L.**	**24 h**	**B.L.**	**24 h**	**B.L.**	**24 h**
Mean (n = 6)	–	–	1.30	1.21	354	369	3750	3610
Precision (%)	–	–	6.8	7.0	3.8	2.7	2.5	4.1
Accuracy (%)	–	–	96.8		92.3		90.3	
C.	**0.5***		**1.25***		**15.0***		**400***	
Mean (n = 6)	0.512		1.24		15.2		378	
Precision (%)	7.2		6.9		2.3		4.6	
Accuracy (%)	102.4		99.2		101.3		94.5	

A. Freeze/thaw stability; B. Ambient temperature stability; C. Autosampler stability (plasmas extract stored at 4°C, reinjection reproducibility). B.L. Baseline.
**Nominal concentration of PH46. #Samples diluted 10-fold prior to extraction and analysis.*

Table 9.
Stability tests (freeze/thaw, ambient temperature & reinjection reproducibility) of PH46 in human plasma.

3. Materials and methods

The research work reported in this article was carried out following the Principles of the Organisation for Economic Co-operation and Development (OECD) of Good Laboratory Practice (GLP) as accepted by international regulatory authorities, including EMA (EU), FDA & EPA (USA) and MHLW, MAFF & METI (Japan).

		−20°C			−80°C	
A.	1.25*	400*	4000*,#	1.25*	400*	4000*,#
Mean (n = 6)	1.23	402	3990	1.18	405	4100
Precision (%)	3.8	4.3	2.5	2.9	1.6	13.9
Accuracy (%)	98.4	100.5	99.8	94.4	101.3	102.5
	−20°C			**−80°C**		
B.	25.0*	1600*	16,000*,#	25.0*	1600*	16,000*,#
Mean (n = 6)	23.1	1400	15,200	23.8	1480	13,800
Precision (%)	10.3	15.0	6.2	12.0	8.2	9.1
Accuracy (%)	92.4	87.5	95.0	95.2	92.5	86.3
C.	**0.5***	**1.25***		**15***	**400**	
Mean (n = 6)	0.544	1.36		16.4	424	
Precision (%)	6.4	2.6		2.5	1.2	
Accuracy (%)	108.8	108.8		109.3	106.0	
D.	**10***	**25***		**100***	**1600**	
Mean (n = 6)	8.76	24.4		103	1460	
Precision (%)	7.5	10.4		10.1	5.3	
Accuracy (%)	87.6	97.6		103.0	91.3	

**Nominal concentration of PH46 (ng/ml for urine and ng/g eq. for faeces). #samples diluted 10-fold prior to extraction and analysis. A. freezing stability (urine); B. freezing stability (faeces); C. reinjection reproducibility (urine); D. reinjection reproducibility (faeces).*

Table 10.
Stability tests (one month storage and reinjection reproducibility) of PH46 in human urine and faeces.

Ethical approval was obtained through Trinity College Dublin which complies with the Council for International Organisations of Medical Sciences' (CIOMS), International Guiding Principles for Biomedical Research.

3.1 Chemical and reagents

PH46A [purity 97.1% with moisture and solvent free; correction factor (purity and salt content): 0.6429] and Compound 1 as IStd (**Figure 1**) were obtained from Trino Therapeutics Ltd. (Ireland). Control human plasma (using lithium heparin as anticoagulant), urine and faeces were obtained from Charles River Laboratories (UK) and stored at −20°C when not in use. All control plasma was mixed and centrifuged prior to use. Control human faeces was homogenised prior to use with addition of deionised H_2O (1:3, faeces:H_2O, *w/v*). HPLC grade solvents and additives, including methanol (MeOH), ACN, H_2O, ammonia solution (28.0–30.0%), acetic acid (AA), acetone, dimethylsulphoxide (DMSO), chloroform ($CHCl_3$), TFA and FA, were purchased commercially between VWR (Ireland), Fisher Scientific (Ireland) and Sigma-Aldrich (Ireland) and were of analytical/HPLC grade or equivalent.

	Baseline	1 M	1 M^{+}	2 M	3 M	4 M	4 M^{+}	5 M
A.								
1.25*								
Mean (n = 6)	1.30	1.06	0.918	1.22	–	1.03	1.01	–
Precision (%)	6.8	5.9	5.8	6.8		5.6	2.9	
Accuracy (%)	n/a	84.8^	73.4^	97.6		82.4^	80.8^	
400*								
Mean (n = 6)	354	321	268	389	–	355	–	–
Precision (%)	3.8	2.9	2.4	2.2		1.2		
Accuracy (%)	n/a	80.3^	67.0^	97.3		88.8		
4000$^{*,\#}$								
Mean (n = 6)	3750	3310	3140	3940	–	3810	–	–
Precision (%)	2.5	2.7	3.5	4.8		1.4		
Accuracy (%)	n/a	82.8^	78.5^	98.5		95.3		
B.								
1.25*								
Mean (n = 6)	1.22	1.19	–	–	1.15	–	–	1.21
Precision (%)	9.2	2.9			3.3			5.7
Accuracy (%)	n/a	95.2			92.0			96.8
400*								
Mean (n = 6)	371	363	–	–	389	–	–	377
Precision (%)	2.1	3.7			1.5			2.8
Accuracy (%)	n/a	90.8			97.3			94.3
4000$^{*,\#}$								
Mean (n = 6)	3820	3640	–	–	3740	–	–	3720
Precision (%)	1.8	1.6			0.7			2.2
Accuracy (%)	n/a	91.0			93.5			93.0

M: month. – : not applicable. A. stability test at −20°C; B. stability test at −80°C.
**Nominal concentration of PH46.* $^{+}$*Repeat timepoint experiment.* $^{\#}$*Samples diluted 10-fold prior to extraction and analysis.* ^*Does not meet acceptance criteria (100 ± 15%).*

Table 11.
Storage stability tests of PH46 in human plasma at −20°C and −80°C.

3.2 Instrumentation and operation conditions

AB Sciex API3000 LC/MS/MS spectrometer system: HPLC pump, vacuum degasser, column oven (Series 200, Perkin Elmer), autosampler (HTS Pal, CTC Analytics) along with data handling system (Analyst Version 1.4.2, AB Sciex) and Laboratory Information Management System (Watson 7.0, Thermo Fisher Scientific) for operations and data analysis. Halo C18 LC column (75 × 2.1 mm, 2.7 μm, HiChrom) and PreFrit Filter guard column (0.5 μm, 6.35 × 1.57 mm, Anachem) were used. Column and autosampler temperatures were 60°C and 4°C, respectively. Mobile phase A: MeOH:AA (100:0.2, *v/v*) and mobile phase B: H_2O:AA (100:0.2, *v/v*). The gradient was 60% A (0 min), 80% A (5.0 min), 100% A (6.0 min), 60% A (6.5 min). Flow rate was 0.3 mL/min with injection volume of 10 µL and run time of 6.5 min. The solvent mixtures as needle wash were H_2O:ACN/TFA (25:75:0.1, *v/v/v*) and H_2O:ACN: FA:TFA (90:10:0.1:0.005, *v/v/v/v*). Sample diluent was MeOH:H_2O:AA (50:50:0.2, *v/v/v*). TurboIonSpray negative ionisation mode was applied to carry out the detection of mass spectrometry. Nitrogen (API3000) was used for nebulizing and drying, with 700°C of ion spray temperature and −4500 V of ion spray voltage. PH46 and IStd ions monitored were 381.10–135.10 (±0.5) and 409.20–164.00 (±0.5) dwell time 200 ms.

3.3 Preparation of CSs and QC samples

The PH46 and IStd primary stock solutions were prepared at 1 mg/mL in ACN: DMSO (50:50, *v/v*). The plasma/urine CSs at concentrations of 0.5, 1, 3.25, 12.5, 50, 150, 450 and 500 ng/mL) were made by serial dilutions of the primary stock in control matrix. For each batch of plasma/urine samples, 200 µL aliquots of the bulk CSs were extract (duplicate) resulting in different concentrations of PH6 within the linear concentration range of the assay. 15 ng/mL of IStd solution was also made from the primary IStd stock solution using a mixture of MeOH:$CHCl_3$ (50:50, *v/v*). The bulk faeces CSs were prepared by serially diluting the stock solution in homogenised control faeces to give 10, 20, 48, 120, 280, 720, 1800 and 2000 ng/g faecal equivalent. For each batch of faeces samples, aliquots (1 mL, equivalent to 250 mg of faecal material) of the bulk CSs were extracted in duplicate to give a range of concentrations of PH46 within the linear range of the assay and a fixed concentration of IStd (60 ng/g faecal equivalent).

Plasma/urine QC samples were prepared in control matrix from the primary PH46 stock solution in similar manner as CSs, to give QC samples at 0.5 (LLOQ), 1.25 (low), 15 (medium) and 400 (high) ng/mL plasma/urine concentrations and aliquots (200 µL) of the bulk QC samples were extracted for analysis. For faeces QC samples, concentrations were made at 10 (LLOQ), 25 (low), 100 (medium) and 1600 (high) ng/mL faecal equivalent, and aliquots (1 mL, equivalent to 250 ng of faecal material) of the bulk QC samples were extracted for analysis. All sample solutions were stored in a freezer set to maintain a temperature of −20°C in dark when not use and brought to RT before analysis. To all weighing, a correction for batch specific purity and a correction for salt content (free acid (382.5)/salt (577.7)) were applied.

3.4 Preparation of control matrix and sample extraction

Control plasma (Lithium Heparin anticoagulant), urine and homogenised faeces (1:3 faecal/H_2O slurry, *w/v* by blending until a smooth consistency was obtained), stored at −20°C when not in use, were removed from the freezer and allowed to thaw at RT. Control matrix (pooled) was vortex mixed and centrifuged (3500 rpm, 4°C & 5 min) prior to use. 200 µL (1 mL in the case of homogenised faeces, equivalent to 250 mg faeces) was added to a clean, dry screw cap glass tube (12 × 75 mm) for DB (control matrix only without PH46/IStd) and SB (control matrix with IStd only) samples. CSs, QC and test samples were removed from the freezer and allowed to thaw at RT and vortex mixed prior to aliquoting. 200 µL of aliquots (1 mL in the case of faeces) of each sample solution were added to clean glass tubes (12 × 75 mm). 50 µL (10 µL in the case of in the case of faeces) of IStd in MeOH:$CHCl_3$ (50:50, *v/v*) at a working concentration of 0.06 µg/mL (1.5 µg/mL) was added to all samples except for the DB samples, where 50 μL (10 μL instead in the case of faeces) of MeOH:$CHCl_3$ (50:50, *v/v*) was added. A further 2 mL of MeOH:$CHCl_3$ mixture (50:50, *v/v*) (4 mL of $CHCl_3$ in the case of faeces) was added to all samples and the tubes were sealed and vortex mixed thoroughly prior to centrifugation (3500 rpm, 5 min, 4°C). The supernatant from all samples (the lower $CHCl_3$ layer in the case of faeces) was transferred to clean tubes, dried under nitrogen at 60°C and then reconstituted in 100 μL of MeOH:H_2O:AA (50:50:0.2, *v/v/v*). The extracts were then vortex-mixed and transferred into plastic matrix tubes before being centrifuged for 5 min at 3500 rpm at 4°C.

3.5 Validation procedures

When the reference standard PH46A was weighed, a correction factor was made for the salt content. Therefore, all peak area measurement and determined concentrations reported in the study were for PH46 (the free acid form). Each batch of samples had matrix DB, matrix SB, CSs, QC and test sample extracts. Duplicate DB and SB samples and CSs at each level were extracted. The CSs which met the acceptance criteria were used to construct the calibration curve. Two replicates were injected: one at the start and one at the end of the run. Concentration order was used for CS injections in each section of the run. QC samples were made in control matrix at three concentrations: low, medium and high ($n \geq 2$ at each level). Where $n = 2$ at each level were prepared, the samples were injected as follows: one low-QC and one medium-QC level samples were injected at the start of the run following the first set of CSs, one Low-QC and one High-QC level samples were injected at the end of the run prior to the second set, and the remaining Medium-QC and High-QC level samples were injected midway through the run. In the case of $n > 2$ at each level were prepared, extra QC samples were appropriately distributed through the run. In order to avoid potential assay carry-over, the injections of solvent or extracted matrix DB samples were made after the high concentration extracts before the injection of low concentration extract.

The acceptance criteria were: (i) at least 75% of the CSs must back-calculate to within 100 ± 15% (plasma and urine assays) or 100 ± 20% (faeces assay) of the nominal concentrations (100 ± 20% at the LLOQ for plasma and urine assays or 100 ± 25% at the LLOQ for faeces assay); (ii) at least 67% of the total number of QC samples in each batch had to be within 100 ± 15% (plasma and urine) or 100 ± 20% (faeces) of the nominal concentrations for the determined concentrations, including at least one QC sample at each concentration had to meet this criterion. Precision was calculated as CV of mean. Accuracy was calculated as mean determined concentration/nominal concentration.

3.5.1 Determination of stability of stored spiking solutions

The stability of the PH46 storing stock solutions in ACN:DMSO (50:50, *v/v*) in a refrigerator set to maintain 4°C was examined by comparing the peak area ratios of the fresh stock solutions with the stock solutions on 200 days storage. The preparation of all stock solutions were performed in the same way. The ULOQ solutions were prepared by diluting the stock solutions using an appropriate diluent. The stability of the IStd storing solutions in ACN:DMSO, (50:50, *v/v*) for the stock solution and MeOH:$CHCl_3$ (50:50, *v/v*) for the working solution, in a refrigerator set to maintain 4° C was also studied by comparing the peak area ratios of the freshly prepared and diluted stock and working solutions with the previous stocks on 250 days storage and previous working solutions on 192 days storage, respectively. PH46 and IStd were considered to be stable if the mean responses (MRs) for the stored solutions were within 100 ± 10% of the MRs of the fresh solutions and ≤ 10% for the precision.

The stability of the PH46 storing stocks at ambient RT was also investigated by comparing the peak area ratios of an aliquot of the stock solution (4°C) against an aliquot of the same stock solution on storage at ambient RT for 24 h. Dilutions were made to both solutions to the ULOQ level with an appropriate diluent. PH46 was considered to be stable at RT when the MRs of the solutions stored at RT were within 100 ± 10% of the MRs from the solutions at 4°C and ≤ 10% for the precision.

3.5.2 Linearity and specificity

For each batch, the calibration curve over 0.5–500 ng/mL (plasma and urine assays) or 10–2000 ng/g (faeces assay) was constructed from PH46:IStd area response ratios plotted against the nominal matrix concentrations of PH46 to determine the optimum regression parameters, using linear regression with $1/x^2$ weighting factor. The matrix concentration of PH46 from each CSs was calculated from the corresponding curve. DB and SB samples were also extracted and analysed; but not included in the regression analysis. For the batch to be acceptable the determined matrix concentration of PH46 for each sample used to construct the calibration curve, had to be 100 ± 15% (plasma and urine assays) or 100 ± 20% (faeces assay) of the nominal matrix concentration (100 ± 20% (plasma and urine assays) or 100 ± 25% (faeces assay) of the nominal matrix concentration at LLOQ). At least 75% (including at least one LLOQ and one ULOQ samples) of the CSs had to meet the above criteria.

The specificity of the assay for PH46 and IStd was determined by extraction and analysis of one DB sample from six independent sources of control matrix, three SB samples in a single source of control matrix and three ULOQ samples (without IStd) in the same source of control matrix as for SBs. If interfering peaks at the retention time of PH46 and/or IStd were noted, these were deemed to be insignificant if the response at the retention time of PH46 in the DB and SB samples was ≤20% of the average analyte response in LLOQ CSs and if the response at the retention time of IStd in DB and ULOQ samples was ≤5% of the IStd response accepted in the calibration curve, including SBs.

3.5.3 Assay recovery and matrix effect

The matrix effects on the plasma assay were determined by extracting replicate (n = 6) samples of control matrix, from six individual sources with one of these sources also presented as haemolysed plasma and spiking appropriate volumes of PH46 and IStd solutions (prepared in MeOH:H_2O:AA (50:50:0.2, *v/v/v*) following extraction. Three replicate matrix effect samples at each of the matrix equivalent concentrations (1.25 and 400 ng/mL) and IStd concentration (15 ng/mL) were generated. Spiking appropriate volumes (as above) of the PH46 and IStd solutions in the same ratio as the extract samples resulted in replicate (n = 3) non-extracted QC samples. The ratio of the MR of replicate samples spiked into matrix to the MR of the non-extracted samples was calculated to determine the MF for PH46 and IStd in each source of matrix. The value of (PH46-MF)/(IStd-MF) from the same source was calculated to determine the IStd-normalised MF. There was deemed to be no matrix effect in the samples when the precision of the IStd-normalised MF (calculated from the six sources) was ≤15% at each level.

The recovery of the plasma assay was investigated following the preparation, extraction and analysis of replicate (n = 3) matrix-effect samples, at low, medium and high levels, from a single matrix source. Replicate (n = 3) extracted samples were prepared following the details in Section 3.5.4 at the same concentration levels (low, medium and high) as the matrix-effect samples. The recoveries of PH46 and IStd were calculated as: MRs in the extracted samples/MRs in the matrix-effect samples.

3.5.4 Intra-batch assay accuracy and precision

The accuracy and precision of intra-batch assay were assessed using replicate (n = 6) QC samples prepared in control matrix at 0.5 (LLOQ), 1.25 (low), 15 (medium) and 400 (high) ng/mL for the plasma and urine assays, and 10 (LLOQ), 25 (low), 100 (medium) and 1600 (high) ng/g faecal equivalent for the faeces assay. The intra-batch accuracy expressed as the mean percentage determined concentration/ nominal concentration. For the plasma and urine assays, the acceptance criteria were expected to be within 100 ± 15% at each concentration level (100 ± 20% at LLOQ level) for all three occasions. For the faeces assay, the criteria for acceptance at each level were within 100 ± 20% (100 ± 25% at the LLOQ level). The intra-batch precision was determined by the CV of the mean determined concentration. The criteria for acceptance should be ≤15% at each level (≤20% at LLOQ level) for all three occasions for the plasma and urine assays or ≤ 20% (≤25% at the LLOQ level) for the faeces assay. The inter-batch assay accuracy and precision were determined on three occasions (on different days). The acceptance criteria at each level were that assay accuracy for all three occasions was within 100 ± 15% (100 ± 20% at the LLOQ level), and that the assay precision for all three occasions was ≤15% (≤20% at the LLOQ level).

3.5.5 Assay carry-over and matrix dilution

Carry-over was assessed by the preparation, extraction and analysis of replicate (n = 2) samples prepared in control matrix at concentrations of 0.5 ng/mL (assay LLOQ) and 500 ng/mL (assay ULOQ). Additional replicate (n = 2) DB samples were also prepared, extracted and analysed. The samples were analysed in the following sequence: ULOQ (x1), DB (x2), LLOQ (x1), ULOQ (x1), solvent samples (MeOH: H_2O:AA, 50:50:0.2, *v/v/v*) (x2) and LLOQ (x1). The assay was deemed to have no carry-over for PH46 when the responses for PH46 in DB and solvent samples were ≤ 20% of the detector responses for PH46 in the next LLOQ samples. The assay was deemed to have no carry-over for IStd if the responses for IStd in DB and solvent samples were ≤ 5% of the detector responses for the IStd in the previous ULOQ samples. A bulk stock (4 mg/mL of PH46 in control plasma/urine or 16 mg/g faecal equivalents in control homogenised faeces) was prepared in control matrix. Replicate (n = 6) QC samples from this stock were diluted 10- and 100-fold with control matrix. Aliquots (200 μL for plasma/urine assays or 1 mL equivalent to 250 mg faecal material for faecal assay) (n = 6 of each dilution factor) were then extracted (nominal concentrations of 400 and 40 ng/mL respectively for plasma/urine assays or 1.6 mg/g and 160 ng/g faecal equivalent respectively for the faecal assay). The determined concentrations were corrected for the dilution factors. Matrix dilution was considered to be acceptable if the assay accuracy was within 100 ± 15% for the plasma/urine assays or 100 ± 20% for the faeces assay, and the assay precision was ≤15% for the urine assay and ≤ 20% for the faeces assay.

3.5.6 Stability experiments

For the following stability experiments, bulk QC samples were prepared at the appropriate low, high and dilution levels for each assay. A 10-fold dilution in control matrix was carried out on the dilution level QC before extraction and analysis.

3.5.6.1 Determination of short-term frozen storage stability and freeze/thaw stability of PH46 in matrix

Six aliquots (200 µL) at each concentration were extracted and analysed immediately to confirm the suitability of the stability samples. The remainder of each bulk was aliquoted into tubes (n = 18 for plasma, n = 48 for urine and n = 46 for faeces) containing a greater volume than required for analysis. Half of the replicates in each matrix (urine and faeces) were stored at −20°C and the other half of the replicates in each matrix were stored at −80°C. The effects of the corresponding stability samples were investigated after at least 1 month storage. The freeze/thaw stability of PH46 in plasma matrix assay was performed by using QCs samples (n = 6) at each concentration subjecting to freeze/thaw cycles (×3) in a freezer set to maintain −20°C (initial freeze cycle 24 h as minimum, freeze cycles 2 and 3 at least 12 h and thaw cycle for one h ± 6 min at RT unprotected from light). At the time point, replicate samples (n = 6) at each concentration and each condition were then extracted and analysed with fresh CSs and QCs. The samples were deemed to be stable if the accuracy was within 100 ± 15% (urine and plasma) or 100 ± 20% (faeces) of the nominal concentration and the CV was ≤15% (urine and plasma) or ≤ 20% (faeces) at each concentration level.

3.5.6.2 Determination of re-injection reproducibility

The accuracy and precision batch for each assay was re-injected, having stored the extracts in an autosampler at 4°C for at least 239 h for plasma extracts, at least 25 days for urine extracts and at least 6.5 days for faeces extracts.

3.5.6.3 Determination of ambient RT stability of PH46 in matrix

Ambient RT stability of PH46 in plasma was assessed on further QCs (n = 6) at each level after being left at ambient temperature (unprotected from light) for 24 h ± 30 min before extraction with fresh CSs and QCs.

3.5.6.4 Determination of extended frozen storage stability of PH46 in matrix

Six aliquots (200 µL) at each concentration were extracted and analysed immediately to show that the stability samples had been suitably prepared. The remainder of each bulk was aliquoted into glass tubes (n ≥ 48) containing a greater volume than required for analysis. The extended frozen storage stability of PH46 in human plasma was investigated after at least one, two and four months at −20°C and the effects of storing samples at −80°C were also assessed after at least one, three and five months. At each time point, replicates (n = 6) at each concentration were extracted and analysed with fresh CSs and QC samples. The samples were deemed to be stable if the accuracy was within 100 ± 15% of the nominal concentration and the CV was ≤15% at each concentration level.

3.6 Data handling, processing and calculations

Analyst® 1.4.2 software was used for data collection during the study. Thermo Fisher Scientific Watson™ 7.0 software was employed to determine the calibration parameters/values, including slope, intercept and coefficient of determination, the mean, standard deviation and accuracy data. Three significant digits were presented for the nominal matrix concentration (CS and QC samples) and the determined concentration results. The calculations of the accuracy and precision data were made from the rounded mean values and from the unrounded determined concentration data and peak area data, respectively, and were displayed to one decimal place. Four significant digits were reported for slopes and intercepts, four decimal places were for coefficients of determination, and six decimal places for instrument responses.

4. Conclusions

In summary, we developed and validated a sensitive and specific bioanalytical method for the determination of PH46, a potential anti-inflammatory bowel disease agent, in human plasma, urine and faeces. A range of testing, including solution stability, specificity, assay linearity, accuracy, precision, recovery, matrix effect, carry-over, dilution effect and stabilities, were established for the matrices. The method meets EMA validation criteria. This method was successfully applied to the clinical pharmacokinetic study of PH46A in human.

Acknowledgements

This work was supported by The Wellcome Trust (grant reference no. 067033/Z/02/A), Enterprise Ireland. The authors would like to acknowledge the contributions of Charles River Laboratories for providing the human plasma (proposal no. 313701) and the technical input throughout this study. The authors also acknowledge NatPro for the funding for APC of this publication.

Conflict of interest

The authors declare no conflict of interest.

Author contributions

Conceptualisation, N.F. and H.S.; investigation, H.S.; funding acquisition, N.F. and H.S.; data curation, G.A.S. and T.Z.; data analysis, T.Z. and G.A.S.; methodology, G.A.S. and T.Z.; data supervision, G.A.S.; writing—original draft, T.Z.; writing—review and editing: T.Z., G.A.S., N.F., H.S. All authors have read and agreed to the published version of the manuscript.

Author details

Tao Zhang[1,2,3*†], Gaia A. Scalabrino[1,3†], Neil Frankish[1,4] and Helen Sheridan[1,3,4*]

1 Trino Therapeutics Ltd, The Tower, Trinity Technology and Enterprise Campus, Dublin, Ireland

2 School of Food Science and Environmental Health, Technological University Dublin, Grangegorman, Dublin, Ireland

3 NatPro Centre, School of Pharmacy and Pharmaceutical Sciences, Trinity College Dublin, Dublin, Ireland

4 School of Pharmacy and Pharmaceutical Sciences, Trinity College Dublin, Dublin, Ireland

*Address all correspondence to: tao.zhang@tudublin.ie; hsheridn@tcd.ie

†These authors contributed equally and should be considered joint first authors.

References

[1] Bai H, Chen X, Zhang L, Dou X. The effect of sulindac, a non-steroidal anti-inflammatory drug, attenuates inflammation and fibrosis in a mouse model of chronic pancreatitis. BMC Gastroenterology. 2012;**12**:115

[2] Prakasham AP, Saxena AK, Luqman S, Chanda D, Kaur T, Gupta A, et al. Synthesis and anticancer activity of 2-benzylidene indanones through inhibiting tubulin polymerization. Bioorganic & Medicinal Chemistry. 2012;**20**(9):3049-3057

[3] Luan F, Cordeiro MN, Alonso N, García-Mera X, Caamaño O, Romero-Duran FJ, et al. TOPS-MODE model of multiplexing neuroprotective effects of drugs and experimental-theoretic study of new 1,3-rasagiline derivatives potentially useful in neurodegenerative diseases. Bioorganic & Medicinal Chemistry. 2013;**21**(7):1870-1879

[4] Melillo B, Liang S, Park J, Schön A, Courter JR, LaLonde JM, et al. Small-molecule CD4-mimics: Structure-based optimization of HIV-1 entry inhibition. ACS Medicinal Chemistry Letters. 2016; **7**(3):330-334

[5] Zhang T, McCabe T, Marzec B, Frankish N, Sheridan H. N-Cycloípentyl-N-(3-oxo-2,3-dihydro-1H-inden-1-yl) acetamide. Acta Crystallographica Section E, Structure Reports Online. 2012;**68**:o958

[6] Zhang T, Paluch K, Scalabrino G, Frankish N, Healy AM, Sheridan H. Molecular structure studies of (1S,2S)-2-benzyl-2,3-dihydro-2-(1H-inden-2-yl)-1H-inden-1-ol. Journal of Molecular Structure. 2015;**1083**:286-299

[7] Frampton CS, Zhang T, Scalabrino GA, Frankish N, Sheridan H. (1S)-1-Phenylethanaminium 4-{[(1S,2S)-1-hydroxy-2,3-dihydro-1H,1'H-[2,2′-biinden]-2-yl]methyl} benzoate. Acta Crystallographica. Section C. 2012;**68**(Pt 8):0323-0326

[8] Sheridan H, Lemon S, Frankish N, McArdle P, Higgins T, James JP, et al. Synthesis and antispasmodic activity of nature identical substituted indanes and analogues. European Journal of Medicinal Chemistry. 1990;**25**(7): 603-608

[9] Sheridan H, Frankish N, Farrell R. Synthesis and antispasmodic activity of analogues of natural pterosins. European Journal of Medicinal Chemistry. 1999; **34**(11):953-966

[10] Sheridan H, Frankish N, Farrell R. Smooth muscle relaxant activity of pterosin Z and related compounds. Planta Medica. 1999;**65**(3):271-272

[11] Frankish N, Farrell R, Sheridan H. Investigation into the mast cell stabilizing activity of nature-identical and synthetic indanones. Journal of Pharmacy and Pharmacology. 2004; **56**(11):1423-1427

[12] Sheridan H, Walsh JJ, Jordan M, Cogan C, Frankish N. A series of 1, 2-coupled indane dimers with mast cell stabilisation and smooth muscle relaxation properties. European Journal of Medicinal Chemistry. 2009;**44**(12): 5018-5022

[13] Sheridan H, Walsh JJ, Cogan C, Jordan M, McCabe T, Passante E, et al. Diastereoisomers of 2-benzyl-2, 3-dihydro-2-(1H-inden-2-yl)-1H-inden-1-ol: Potential anti-inflammatory agents. Bioorganic & Medicinal Chemistry Letters. 2009;**19**(20):5927-5930

[14] Chan K, Frankish N, Zhang T, Ece A, Cannon A, O'Sullivan J, et al. Bioactive indanes: Insight into the bioactivity of indane dimers related to the lead anti-inflammatory molecule PH46A. Journal of Pharmacy and Pharmacology. 2020; **72**(7):927-937

[15] Frankish N, Sheridan H. 6-(methylamino)hexane-1,2,3,4,5-pentanol 4-(((1S,2S)-1-hydroxy-2,3-dihydro-1H,1'H-[2,2-biinden]-2-yl) methyl)benzoate (PH46A): A novel small molecule with efficacy in murine models of colitis. Journal of Medicinal Chemistry. 2012;**55**(11): 5497-5505

[16] Scalabrino GA, Zhang T, Frankish N, Sheridan H. Bioactive indanes: Development and validation of an LC-MS/MS bioanalytical method for the determination of PH46A, a new potential anti-inflammatory agent, in dog and rat plasma and its application to a pharmacokinetic study in dog. Journal of Pharmaceutical and Biomedical Analysis. 2020;**179**:113011

[17] Zhang T, Scalabrino G, Frankish N, Sheridan H. Bioactive Indanes: Comparative in vitro metabolism study of PH46A, a new potential anti-inflammatory agent and biosynthesis of its primary metabolite PH132. Journal of Drug Metabolism & Toxicology. 2018;**9** (2):239

[18] Zhang T, Scalabrino G, Frankish N, Sheridan H. Bioactive Indanes: Proof of concept study for enantioselective synthetic routes to PH46A, a new potential anti-inflammatory agent. Molecules. 2018;**23**(7):1503

[19] Cumming GR, Zhang T, Scalabrino G, Frankish N, Sheridan H. Investigation of the stereoselective synthesis of the Indane dimer PH46A, a new potential anti-inflammatory agent. Organic Process Research and Development. 2017;**21**(12):1972-1979

[20] ISRCTN registry [Internet]. 2023. Available from: www.isrctn.com/ISRCTN90725219

[21] FDA. Guidance for Industry: Bioanalytical Method Validation. Washington D.C., USA: US Department of Health and Human Services. Food and Drug Administration. Center for Drug Evaluation and Research; Center for Veterinary Medicine; 2001

[22] EMA. Guideline on Bioanalytical Method Validation. London, UK: European Medicines Agency, Science Medicines Health, Committee for Medicinal Products for Human Use (CHMP); 2011